Be a Survivor™

Your Guide to Breast Cancer Treatment

Seventh Edition

Be a Survivor™
Your Guide to Breast Cancer Treatment — 7th ed.

Vladimir Lange, M.D.

For information contact:

Lange Productions,
11331 Skyline Drive, Santa Ana CA 92705   714-389-5532
www.LangeProductions.com
marketing@LangeProductions.com
-
ISBN 978-0-692-17724-2

First printing, Seventh edition, September 2018
Second printing, Seventh edition, December 2019

A CIP record for this book is available from the Library of Congress.

Printed in the United States of America

Be a Survivor™

Your Guide to Breast Cancer Treatment

Seventh Edition

VLADIMIR LANGE, M.D.

Lange
PRODUCTIONS

*To Mandy,
Chad, and Christy*

Credits

Graphic Artists:
Christina Lange
Vladimir Lange, MD
Nigel Lizaranzu
Sam Yano

Contributing Writer:
Christina Lange

Photography:
Micaela Bensko Photography
Vladimir Lange, MD
Chad Lange, MD
Erin McFarland Photography
Amy Opfell, MD
Alexandra Scott, Scott Video Productions

Reviewers:
Nina Clapp, RN
William H. Goodson III, MD
Candace Moorman, MPH
Carol Reed

Table of Contents

ACKNOWLEDGMENTS   1

INTRODUCTION TO THE SEVENTH EDITION   3

A Thirty-Year Retrospective   3
How to Use This Book   5
Breast Cancer Facts to Remember   6

CHAPTER 1 - FACING BREAST CANCER   7

Understanding Your Feelings   8
Sharing the News   9
Assembling Your Support Network   16
Gathering Information   19
Overview of Treatment Options   20

CHAPTER 2 - BREAST CANCER BASICS   23

Breast Anatomy and Function   23
How Breasts Grow and Change   25
What is Breast Cancer?   25
Types of Breast Cancer   28
How Cancer Spreads   30

CHAPTER 3 - DIAGNOSIS AND STAGING   31

Diagnosis   31
Tumor Testing   32
Genomic Testing   33
The Pathology Report   34
Additional Tests   34
Staging   36

CHAPTER 4 - SURGERY   **39**

Lumpectomy   40
Is Lumpectomy Right for Me?   43
Mastectomy   45
Recovery After Mastectomy   48
Exercises After Mastectomy   50
Is Mastectomy Right for Me?   51
Lumpectomy or Mastectomy?   52
Axillary Lymph Node Dissection   54
Sentinel Lymph Node Biopsy   56

CHAPTER 5 - RECONSTRUCTION   **57**

Choosing a Plastic Surgeon   58
Reconstruction Options   58
Reconstruction With Implants   59
Reconstruction With Your Own Tissues   62
Which is Right for Me?   67
External Breast Forms   68

CHAPTER 6 - RADIATION THERAPY   **69**

What is Radiation Therapy?   69
External Beam Radiation Therapy   70
How Treatment is Given   70
Side Effects of External Beam Radiation Therapy   72
Brachytherapy   73
Intraoperative Radiation Therapy, IORT   73

CHAPTER 7 - CHEMOTHERAPY   **75**

What is Chemotherapy?   76
How Chemotherapy Works   76
How Chemotherapy is Given   77
Side Effects of Chemotherapy   79
Other Side Effects   86
Common Chemotherapy Drugs   88
Do you need chemotherapy   89

CHAPTER 8 - HORMONE THERAPY   **91**

How Does Hormone Therapy Work?   92
Side Effects of Hormone Therapy   94
Who Should Be Treated?   94

CHAPTER 9 - TARGETED THERAPY   **95**

What are Targeted Therapies   95
Herceptin   95
The Future   97

CHAPTER 10 - COMPLEMENTARY AND ALTERNATIVE THERAPIES   **98**

Complementary Therapies   99
Alternative Treatments   103

CHAPTER 11 - DCIS   **104**

What is DCIS?   104
Mastectomy or Lumpectomy?   105
Radiation Therapy or Not?   105
Treatment of DCIS   106
Your Team   106

CHAPTER 12 - CLINICAL TRIALS   **107**

How are Trials Conducted?   108
Participating in a Trial   109
Is a Trial Right for Me?   110

CHAPTER 13 - LIFE AFTER CANCER   **111**

Emotional Recovery   111
Clinical Depression   113
Physical Recovery   114
Intimacy and Sexuality   117
Side Effects of Treatment   117
Fertility   118
Resuming Sexual Activity   119
Single After Breast Cancer   120
Being a Young Survivor   122
New Beginnings   123
Getting Involved   124
Recommendations for Your Family Members   124
Genetic Testing   125

Chapter 14 - A Guide for Your Partner   **126**

What is Breast Cancer?   127
Understanding Your Feelings   127
What Do I Do Now?   129
What She Needs from You   130
Meeting Your Own Needs   135

Chapter 15 - Advanced Breast Cancer   **138**

Recurrent Breast Cancer   138
Treatment of Advanced / Metastatic Breast Cancer   139
Coping with Advanced Breast Cancer   141

Glossary   **142**

Questions to Ask Your Healthcare Providers   **146**

Index   **157**

Notes to Self   **162**

My Healthcare Team   **163**

CONSULTANTS FOR *BE A SURVIVOR*

**This book was developed with the invaluable assistance
of the following leading experts:**

Terri Ades, R.N., Ph.D.
Leslie Botnick, M.D.
R. James Brenner, M.D., J.D.
Kristin Brill, M.D.
Aman Buzdar, M.D.
Nina Clapp, R.N., M.S.N., C.B.C.N., C.N.-B.N.
Cathy Coleman, R.N., O.C.N.
Helen Crothers, M.S.W.
Barbara Fowble, M.D.
William H. Goodson, III, M.D.
Soram Singh Khalsa, M.D.
Lydia Komarnicky, M.D.
Gail Lebovic, M.D.
Joshua Levine, M.D.
Silvana Martino, D.O.
Stephen Mathes, M.D.
Shirley McKenzie, R.N., P.H.N.
Candace Moorman, M.P.H.
Juliann Reiland, M.D.
Christy A. Russell, M.D.
Karen Schmitt, R.N.
Melvin Silverstein, M.D.
Barbara L. Smith, M.D., Ph.D.
David Spiegel, M.D.
Lisa Summerlot, R.N., O.C.N.
Marilou Terpenning, M.D.
Victor Vogel, M.D.
Deane Wolcott, M.D.

THANK YOU...

...to the survivors and their loved ones for sharing their stories.
Your insight will enlighten, and your words will inspire,
those who follow you on this journey.

ACKNOWLEDGMENTS

This book is based on three decades of professional experience creating educational programs about breast cancer, and on my personal experience dealing with breast cancer as the husband of a survivor.

A list of the names of all those who helped me, encouraged me, and taught me during these years would be longer than the book itself. I thank all of them for their time and kind support.

Several of them deserve special gratitude.

My most sincere thanks go to my valued consultants, recognized experts in their fields, who contributed their time and knowledge to make this book informative, accurate, and up-to-date. It is particularly gratifying that two of them, William Goodson and David Spiegel, are my friends and classmates from Harvard Medical School days. Bill reviewed the manuscript from cover to cover, with surgical precision, spotting areas that needed enhancement.

Five of the consultants stand out over the years in how much they contributed of their extensive experience.

Thirty years ago oncology nurse Lisa Summerlot helped write the scripts and overcome the production red tape for many of the video programs on which this book was based.

Karen Schmitt, breast cancer nurse, reviewed the entire opus before publication, mercilessly pointing out where my writing did not measure up.

Twenty years ago Candace Moorman, then head of the Breast Cancer Detection Section at the Department of Health Services, challenged me by announcing that the world did not need another breast cancer book. Then she rewarded me by admitting that she wished she had this book back when she was diagnosed with breast cancer herself.

More recently, dear friend and innovative oncoplastic breast surgeon Juliann Reiland offered a new perspective on what patients could and should expect from their oncoplasty-trained surgeons, and urged me to create a web-based version of the book.

And for the Sixth Edition, Nina Clapp, Breast Nurse Navigator, joined the team and contributed the fine details that made the book even more relevant to patients.

Thank you! Each of you made the book better.

I also want to thank the survivors and their families, who gave freely of their time and candidly shared their stories.

My deep gratitude to Carol Reed who contributes her boundless energy to keep this book within the sights of those who could most benefit from it.

My love and gratitude to our children, Chad and Christy, for always being there for me, for their Mom, and for each other. And most of all, my love and admiration to Mandy, who has survived her battle with breast cancer and remains in my life as a shining beacon, a powerful inspiration, and a valued critic.

Introduction to the Seventh Edition

A Thirty-Year Retrospective

More than a quarter of a century has gone by since my wife Mandy and I heard the words, "It is cancer." The following hours and days felt like years. Endless years filled with fear of death, and confusion about choices.

Bravely, she powered through the mastectomies, and the chemo, and the delayed reconstructions. And she lived to attend—healthy and vibrant—the landmark events that we thought she would never see: our son's graduation from medical school and his marriage, the international art exhibits curated by our daughter, and the birthdays and the Thanksgiving feasts.

Mandy's breast cancer experience has helped us focus on the things that are truly important in life, and overlook the daily nuisances that have no significance in one's ultimate happiness. "I use the good china every day," Mandy jokes.

Why the Book — *Be a Survivor*?

Despite the fact that both of us are physicians, we were totally overwhelmed by the the torrent of information that was thrown at us on the day the diagnosis was announced. In medical school, we had learned about radiation therapy, chemotherapy, surgery... Yet during the initial meeting with our healthcare team, we sat there, wondering whether these people were speaking Greek or Latin. It was weeks before we were able to unravel all the details and ramifications, and begin deciding on a course of treatment.

The experience led to creating *Be a Survivor – Your Guide to Breast Cancer Treatment* – a book that I hope will help you and your loved ones do a better job of understanding what you are facing, and participate in your treatment and recovery.

The book differs from many others in that it is not a single specialist's narrow point of view. Instead, it is a balanced, objective presentation of the latest information, developed in consultation with dozens of top experts in various fields. Their combined wisdom will provide you with a more balanced overview.

New Venues

This year *Be a Survivor* is going east. Far east. My good friend and colleague Ernie Bodai, a renowned breast surgeon and the creator of the internationally used "Breast Cancer Stamp" has spearheaded the formation of Health Interconnect China-America (HICA), along with his great friend and business partner Renjie Yuan, an organization dedicated to building the bridge linking healthcare between the USA and China, and taking the best health care practices from the USA to China. He has chosen *Be a Survivor* as an important piece for the Health Information Platform that HICA is building in China specifically related to breast, lung, colorectal, and prostate cancers.

All of us are excited to see this valuable book now translated and distributed half-way around the globe.

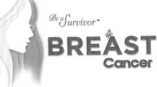

乳腺的结构、功能及发育

作者: Dr. Vladimir Lange

乳房的解剖和功能

首先让我们了解一下乳房的结构和功能。诸如"淋巴结"和"小叶"等术语可能对患者来说比较陌生，但它们将帮助患者更好地理解乳腺癌治疗。

虽然乳房一般呈圆形或泪珠状，但从锁骨到胸线，胸骨到腋窝都存在乳腺组织。这就是为什么在乳腺自检或医生做临床乳腺检查时需要对整个区域进行检查的原因。

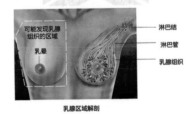

可能发现乳腺组织的区域

乳晕

淋巴结
淋巴管
乳腺组织

乳腺区域解剖

乳房由嵌在脂肪和纤维组织中可以分

Photo courtesy of
HICA Health Information Platform Team

How To Use This Book

The book is organized in the sequence that mirrors your path through treatment and recovery.

First, I've provided a few suggestions on how to come to grips with your feelings about what you were just handed, so you can think and evaluate the facts. There are tips on what to tell your children, family, and co-workers about your diagnosis, and how to assemble a network of support.

Next is an overview of breast cancer treatment. *If you only read one section in this book, make sure it's this one.* It will help you understand how the different aspects of your treatment fit together, so you can see your options more clearly.

The majority of the book consists of detailed information about various treatments, including new developments. There is information on complementary treatments, such as relaxation, visualization, and acupuncture, which may be valuable additions to your battle with cancer.

The book also will help you make a smooth transition from treatment to recovery, both emotionally and physically. It will show you how to follow-up with your doctor, and how to keep yourself healthy.

There is an important chapter devoted to your partner—husband, boyfriend or special man or woman in your life. It not only teaches them how to provide support for you, but also speaks directly to the needs of your partner during this time.

Each chapter includes lists of questions you might want to ask your health-care professionals. For your convenience, these questions are repeated at the end of the book. You can tear out the pages, or take the whole book with you on office visits to help you communicate more effectively.

Let us hope that the day will come when your daughters, and ours, will find this book, and all other books on the topic, "out of print."

We wish you a speedy recovery.

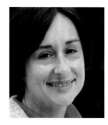

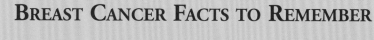
BREAST CANCER FACTS TO REMEMBER

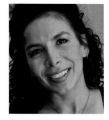

- Breast cancer is not a death sentence—98% of those diagnosed early are **successfully treated**.

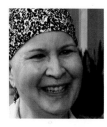

- Breast cancer can often be treated with **breast-conserving surgery**—preserving the natural appearance of the breast.

- Excellent options for **oncoplastic reconstruction** are available if a mastectomy is necessary.

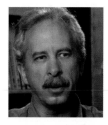

- Today's **genomic testing** can help your medical team design a treatment course taylored to your spcific cancer.

- In most cases there is **no need to rush** your decisions. Take time to learn as much as you can, and to decide what choices are best for you.

- A **positive attitude** and active participation will improve the outcome of your treatment. Resolve that you will survive this challenge.

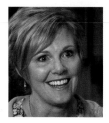 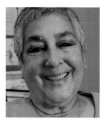 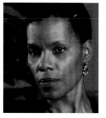 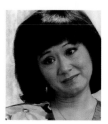 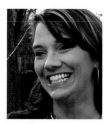

CHAPTER 1

FACING BREAST CANCER

"You have breast cancer."

These may be the most frightening words you've ever heard. You may feel scared, angry, crushed—or in complete denial. And you will have no idea how to begin dealing with your problem.

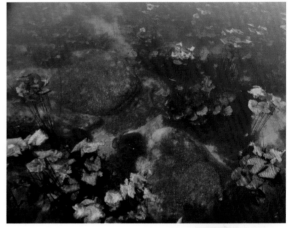

First of all, realize that a diagnosis of breast cancer is not a death sentence. Breast cancer is a very treatable disease, and survival rates today are higher than ever before. There are millions of women who have been handed the same diagnosis many years ago, and are still leading happy, productive lives.

The best approach you can take is to resolve, right now, that you will do everything you can to be successful in your battle against breast cancer. Tell yourself that losing this battle is simply not an option. This positive attitude will be your best ally.

On the following pages we will discuss the initial steps you need to take to reclaim control over the situation:

- Understand your feelings
- Decide how, when, and with whom to share the news
- Assemble a support network
- Gather the information you need
- Actively participate in planning your treatment.

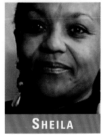

SHEILA

When I heard the doctor say "breast cancer" it was like going underwater. Everything started to move in slow motion, and I couldn't hear anything more. Only when I got to my bedroom, only then I started to cry.

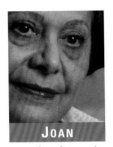

JOAN

When you get that diagnosis, go ahead and cry your eyes out. Cry your eyes out right then, so that you're not bottling up that emotion. It's so terrifying, that for a while you feel as though you're in a fog, and that if you come out of this fog, something terrible is going to happen. So, cry it, vent it, talk it out, and then find out what you can do to help yourself.

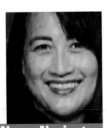

NINA-Nurse Navigator

Other stressors in your life will come together to make things even more difficult. A cancer diagnosis will help you put things in perspective. Setting priorities is a valuable life skill that is never too late to learn.

UNDERSTANDING YOUR FEELINGS

Learning that you have breast cancer is an experience that is probably unlike any other in your life. Don't try to suppress the turmoil that you are experiencing. Cry, get angry, shout. Show whatever emotion helps you, because there is no right or wrong response, and you are entitled to feel whatever you are feeling.

The first few weeks after your diagnosis may be the hardest to handle. On some days, questions like "Will I die?" or "Will my husband still love me?" will invade your mind and incapacitate you. On other days, you will be overcome with joy just to hear a single piece of good news. This emotional roller coaster is difficult to manage. Don't be too hard on yourself if your emotions slip out of your control every once in a while. You don't need to be a superwoman in perfect balance all the time.

Cancer or not, you most likely have other stressors in your life that will compound the challenge. Family obligations. Work deadlines. Holiday plans. Paying bills and cleaning the house and driving the kids... Take a step back and evaluate your priorities. Let some things go, so you can concentrate on the most important--your health.

Find someone you can talk to about what you are experiencing. This should be a mature, well-adjusted person who can listen without passing judgment. Very close friends or family members may be too involved in the situation.

It may be best to speak to someone who is more objective and doesn't have a need to "make it all better." For example, another woman who had breast cancer, or an organized group of breast cancer survivors.

In addition, don't be embarrassed to seek professional help. Counseling can help you come to grips with your feelings, so you can start on the road to recovery.

Most importantly, take a deep breath and don't feel pressured to get everything under control. Typically, breast cancer is a slow growing cancer, and you have weeks or even months to make treatment decisions.

SHARING THE NEWS

Telling Your Partner

In a misguided attempt to protect your loved one, you may try to hide your emotions from him. Don't. It is far better to involve your partner as soon as possible, so the two of you can find strength in each other, and learn from the beginning how you can work as a team in the weeks and months to come.

Try to remember that your husband, boyfriend or partner probably will be affected by your diagnosis as much as you. In some ways his challenge may be particularly difficult because he will have to manage his own emotions, and at the same time shoulder the task of being your key supporter.

Faced with the news many men will feel helpless, and respond by withdrawing or getting angry. Realize that this behavior does not indicate a loss of love, only an extreme frustration. You may need to take on the added burden of helping him help you.

Couples may have difficulty adjusting to the role changes that are sometimes necessary. A partner who was responsible for only part of the daily activities may now become the sole breadwinner and homemaker, preparing dinner, changing the bedding and dressings, and providing companionship and emotional support. The sheer weight of these responsibilities can be overwhelming.

You can help by communicating your needs clearly. "I would love it if you..." will be far better for both of you than some unstated wish left unfulfilled.

A partner's concern or fears can affect your sexual relationship. Some may worry that physical intimacy will harm the person who has cancer. Others may fear that they might "catch" the cancer or be affected by the drugs. Many of these issues can be cleared up by open communications.

It is normal for you to lose desire for your mate for a while as other concerns overshadow your sexual life. Both you and your partner should feel free to discuss this with each other, as well as with your doctor, nurse, or counselor who can give you the information and the reassurance you need.

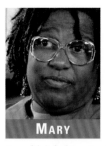

MARY

I couldn't believe it. The last thing I expected to hear was that I had breast cancer. I couldn't have cancer. It was impossible for me to have cancer, because I had all these people to take care of. At my job, I couldn't afford to be sick.

QUESTIONS TO ASK YOUR DOCTOR:

What should I tell my loved ones about my condition?

May I bring members of my family, or a friend, to talk to you directly?

Can you refer me to a counselor or to a support group specializing in breast cancer issues?

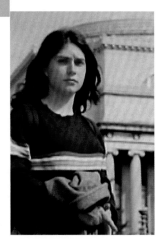

ONE GIRL'S STORY

With the benefit of a thirty-year hindsight, my wife and I feel that we should have handled our communications with our children better. We "protected" them by presenting a rosy picture. It wasn't until years later that we realized the turmoil that our daughter went through during her Mom's treatment. Here is a school essay she wrote as an eleven-year-old. She didn't show it to us until she went off to college.

My father's face is red. A plate of blackened hamburgers is trembling in his hands. I am looking up at his thick, wrinkled forehead as his mouth opens and closes, spilling angry words: "How could you be so careless? Didn't you realize they were burning?" I do not offer any explanation about my carelessness. I just look down at my sneakers and moan.

There is a deafening crash as my father slams the plate of burned food onto our dining room table. My father, my mother, my teenage brother and I slide noiselessly into our chairs. I can feel hot anger burning at the top of my stomach and shooting up into my throat. I strain to hold back the tears, but the liquid collects on my eyelashes, forming droplets that slowly pull themselves down my cheeks.

"Why are you crying?" My father's voice is louder than he expects it to be. The look on his face tells me that he knows I am not crying over burned hamburgers. He knows exactly why I am crying. He would cry those same frustrated tears if his ego would let him.

I am crying because my mother has cancer. It is the third month of her chemotherapy; the third month we have had to pretend that our family is still as strong as it ever was, that my mother's illness is just a temporary setback.

But tonight I am tired of not being able to be a normal eleven-year-old. I am tired of telling my mother that everything is fine, that she doesn't have to be at my soccer game, that it is OK if she is too sick to eat a piece of my birthday cake. It is no longer fine. Our family cannot survive without my mother. It does not matter that my brother had learned to do laundry while my father goes to PTA meetings and I teach myself how to cook. We cannot bear to think that my mother may die, but we cannot hide the fact that we are thinking it.

"Why are you crying?" My father's words are still reverberating in my brain as I search for a safe place to stare so I do not have to face the sadness in the room. I hear a tiny sound, a low whimper escaping from my mother's side of the table. I glance over at her and watch her hunched shoulders moving rhythmically up and down as she fidgets with the tablecloth. She lifts her pale face and looks around the dining room as if she too is wondering where the sound is coming from. Her eyelids are dark red and tears are slipping effortlessly down her face.

It is the first time I have seen my mother cry. I want to look away, but I keep staring. My mother shakes her head slowly, as if she is scolding herself for revealing the pain she has been harboring underneath her confident exterior.

"Oh God, I'm so sorry." The words come tumbling from my mouth. "I'm so sorry, I'm so sorry." I keep vomiting the words. I run to my mother's side, frantic, hoping I can get to her fast enough to return her to the moment before she began suffering. "I'm sorry, Mommy. I'm sorry." I hug her tighter than I ever have before, letting her hair stick to my wet cheek. "I'm so sorry." The words are not even mine anymore. They are escaping from a place in my body that I never knew existed. I am not thinking about anything else, about what my father and brother must be thinking, about what it will be like after this moment. "I'm sorry..."

I'm sorry that I've been selfish, sorry that I got mad when you weren't excited about my report card, sorry I refused to go with you to your first dose of chemotherapy, sorry that I laughed at your new wig, sorry that I ran away when you threw up in the kitchen sink. I'm sorry I didn't know how you were suffering.

I am holding my mother's trembling body. I rest my chin in the crevasse of her shoulder the way I used to when she knelt down to hug me. The room and its contents no longer exist. My mother and I are alone, clinging to each other, and I am wishing that I could heal her. I press my lips to her ear and whisper, "Mommy, please don't die."

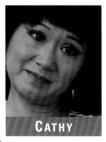

CATHY

I knew that my surgery was just a few days away. And I looked down at my body and at this right breast and I said, "I'm proud of you. You're beautiful. But I am very sorry, you have to go, because you're not my friend any-more." I'm glad I did that. I'm glad that I had made my peace with it.

NINA-Nurse Navigator

Some children have friends whose parents have cancer, and information about their experience may spill over and color their thoughts of what may happen to you. Point out to them that no two cancers are alike.

Telling Your Children

This is one of the more challenging tasks you and your partner will have to handle.

Your first impulse may be to attempt to shield your children from pain by withholding information. Don't underestimate their insight. Children's ability to pick up signals is greater than most people realize, and trying to keep a complex situation such as cancer a secret, is practically impossible. More than likely, they will sense that all is not well, and wander away imagining horrors far worse than reality. The next day they will get a dose of misinformation from their classmates, which will only fuel their fears.

A much better approach is a simple and straightforward explanation. But the explanation must be geared to each child's age and ability to under-stand.

For example, a kindergartener may only be able to grasp the fact that you are sick, and for a while you will need treatment, and may not always be able to play with him.

A high-schooler may be ready to know the exact details of the expected treatment, as well as hear your thoughts and fears.

The discussion must also be well-timed. News that you have cancer may be best delivered after the finals are over, or after the long-planned family holiday.

In all communications, conveying the impression that you are comfortable and that you trust them, will help them deal with the situation.

At any age, children may have difficulty coping with cancer in a parent. Some fear the loss of the parent or begin to imagine their own death. This can play havoc with all aspects of their lives—from school performance, to sleep patterns, to social contacts.

In addition to this upheaval, children often are asked to "play quietly", to perform extra tasks, or to be considerate of others' moods. Some of these demands may far exceed their maturity and understanding.

Younger children may resent lost attention. Teenagers can feel torn between expressing independence and a need to remain close to the sick parent. Discipline problems can arise.

Parents may not have the emotional energy to provide the usual support, love, and authority. It may help if a favorite relative or family friend can devote extra time and attention to the children to help maintain normal family routines as much as possible. Events like trips to the zoo are important, but so is helping with homework, or attending the basketball awards banquet.

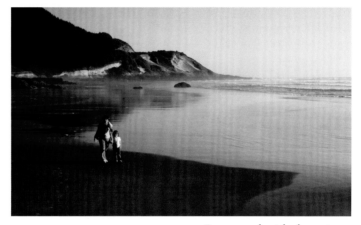

Learn to cherish the quiet moments of togetherness

Remember, breast cancer does not need to be a totally negative experience. Instead, it can serve as a tool that will help your family grow stronger and be more united.

Tips for better communications with children

• Wait until you and your partner have your emotions under some control—perhaps a day or two after the diagnosis.

• Start with a simple statement, adjusted for age and understanding level. For example, "The doctor found a lump in Mommy's breast. It is called cancer, and needs to be taken out..."

• Encourage them to ask questions, and answer them truthfully. Be ready for questions that reflect their fear of being abandoned.

• Involve them by assigning tasks that will make them feel like they are contributing to your recovery. This is especially important for younger children, who may feel responsible for your illness.

• Never underestimate your children's insight, or their ability to gather information and misinformation on their own.

NINA-Nurse Navigator

Talk about boundaries. Remind everyone that the information is not to be shared on social media. You don't want a careless tweet to prompt a slew of calls that you are not ready to answer.

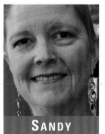

SANDY

Probably the worst part early on was noticing my friends' reaction to my diagnosis. I noticed that some of them stopped calling, stopped e-mailing. I think they were probably afraid that I was in bed, dying... So I created a blog to keep everybody informed.

Telling Your Family

The people who are close to you also will be affected by your news. They too may need to be angry, cry, and express their emotions. It's a natural part of adjusting to your diagnosis. It will help both you and them to talk openly about each other's feelings. Open communication from the start will go a long way toward strengthening the bonds with your loved ones, and securing the support you'll need.

Sometimes the "extended family" can be just too "extended" or too expressive. Their combined concerns can be overwhelming, and may have a negative effect on you. Feel free to limit the lines of communication with relatives who drain, rather than replenish, your energy. Remember, you are the one in charge, and this is the time when you need unwavering support.

Dealing with Friends and Others

Some friends will deal well with your illness and will provide gratifying support. Some will be unable to cope with the possibility of your death, and will disappear from your life. Most will want to help, but may be unsure of how to go about it, and will be waiting for clues from you about where to begin.

You may have to be the one who takes the initiative in reestablishing contact. Reach out to those who don't call. Make specific requests for simple things—to run an errand, prepare a meal, come for a visit. No one who is healthy can imagine how much they will be appreciated if they do nothing but pick up a few things off the floor for a woman who may not be able to bend down for a few days after surgery. These small acts bring friends back into contact and help them feel useful and needed.

When it comes to conversational topics, bear in mind that people who don't have experience dealing with cancer may have no idea what is acceptable. "Isn't it too personal to ask about her breast reconstruction?" or "Should I pretend nothing happened?" or "How do I discuss her fears with her, without making things worse?" Help them by being the first to bring up whatever subject you want to discuss.

Beyond the immediate circle of people who are close to you, no one is entitled to have information you don't want to give out.

Dealing with Employers

At work, you may encounter discrimination on the grounds that people who have cancer take too many sick days, are poor insurance risks, or will make co-workers uncomfortable. Reassure them that once your treatment is over, you will be able to resume your work as before, and are not likely to have unexpected sick days any more frequently than your co-workers.

Needing to work to pay the bills, and taking time off to deal with cancer is a stressful combination. Keep an open line of communications with your Human Resources department or your employer. Under Federal law, most employers cannot discriminate against disabled workers, including people with cancer. These laws apply to Federal employers, employers that receive Federal funds, and private companies with 25 or more employees.

If you are applying for a job with a government agency or a firm with government contracts and believe you did not get the job because of your cancer, you can file a complaint with the Department of Justice. If you believe you were discriminated against by a private employer, you should file your complaint with the closest regional office of the Equal Employment Opportunities Commission.

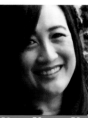

NINA-Nurse Navigator

Friends who disappear aren't necessarily bad friends. They just may feel uncomfortable dealing with your illness, or be reminded of their own vulnerability. Try to keep this in perspective and don't give up good relationships.

Find out more about your rights

• The Cancer Legal Resource Center provides information and education about cancer-related legal issues to the public through its national telephone assistance line.

• Your state's Department of Labor Office of Civil Rights.

• The National Coalition for Cancer Survivorship founded by and for cancer survivors, offers information and limited attorney referrals.

• Regional or national offices of the Civil Liberties Union.

• Your representative's or senator's office has information about Federal and State laws. If you are not sure who represents your district, call your local library.

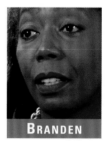

BRANDEN

Develop a really good working relationship with the physicians who are treating you, and let your feelings be known. This is your time. Make sure that everybody is on your team, and don't be afraid to speak up for yourself.

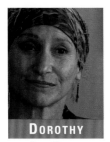

DOROTHY

My group really offers me an opportunity to share my truest feelings, my most private feelings, and my greatest fears in a place where there's support, caring, friendship, and the courage of other people leading you forward.

QUESTIONS TO ASK YOUR DOCTOR:

Can you give me the name of a breast cancer expert who can give me a second opinion?

Could you forward my chart, test results, and my biopsy slides to the doctor who is going to give me a second opinion?

ASSEMBLING YOUR SUPPORT NETWORK

One of your first steps should be to establish a network of people who can help you. This network will center on a solid team of healthcare professionals, and include your loved ones and perhaps a peer support group.

Your Healthcare Team

Cancer is a complicated disease and no single physician can be an expert in all aspects of the treatment. Developing a treatment plan is a complex task that will involve a number of healthcare professionals—a real team of experts—who will give you their recommendations regarding surgery, chemotherapy, radiation and a variety of other issues.

Most hospitals and cancer centers already have such teams of breast cancer experts, called *multidisciplinary* teams. If yours doesn't, the National Cancer Institute, the American Cancer Society, Susan G. Komen for The Cure, or the Breast Cancer Network of Strength have resources that will help you find healthcare professionals to add to your team, or to give you a second opinion.

One of the key people in your network will be the nurse navigator. She will be the person who will guide you through the treatment process, explaining the need for procedures, clarifying issues, setting up appointments and taking your calls when you need to just talk.

Getting a Second Opinion

The treatment of your breast cancer is probably the most important issue you will ever face. For your own peace of mind, now and in the future, consider getting a second opinion. You are entitled to evaluate all your options, and no competent healthcare provider will object to your listening to another viewpoint.

Before your second opinion appointment, be sure to have all your pertinent records either in hand, or sent in from your primary team. These should include all mammograms, other imaging tests, biopsy results, and consultants' notes. Without these, your second opinion will be delayed.

Changing Doctors

Sometimes you may find that one of your physicians seems abrupt, aloof, and uncaring, or fails to convince you of his competence. If this creates a barrier, let the physician know you wish to see someone else. The physician is probably as aware as you are that a good relationship has not been established, and will be happy to transfer your records to another.

But remember, a decision to change physicians should be based on reality and not on a quest to find a doctor who will promise a cure, or guarantee to relieve all your fears.

Friends and Family

Your loved ones will provide the emotional support and closeness you need, and help you sort out facts and fears.

Try to select one person—your husband, partner, or best friend—who will accompany you when you meet with your doctors or go to your treatments. This companion can help you ask questions, remember information, or write down instructions.

He or she can become the center of your support network, acting as your sounding board, helping you to evaluate information and to make decisions, coordinating support from friends and family, and at times shielding you from excessive attention.

Support Groups

One of the most beneficial things you can do is join a support group. Support groups are groups of people who meet regularly, under the guidance of a trained facilitator, to discuss the participants' concerns.

Programs are organized in a variety of ways. Some groups meet only a few times; others are long-term, enabling members to work through problems. Some are composed of people with

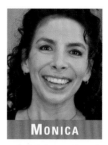

MONICA

I didn't buy what the first two surgeons said - that I couldn't have an expander reconstruction. Finally, I found one who said she could do it. And the result? I have a lovely breast I am proud of...

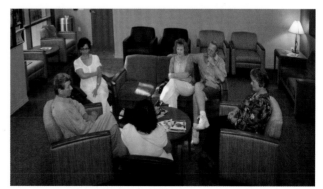

Support groups offer a friendly setting to discuss your concerns.

SPECIALISTS WHO MAY BE INVOLVED IN YOUR TREATMENT:

- **Anesthesiologist:** administers drugs or gasses which put you to sleep before surgery.

- **Breast Surgeon:** will do the initial operation on the cancer, with or without oncoplastic techniques.

- **Clinical Nurse Specialist:** a nurse with training in a specific area, such as post-operative care, chemotherapy, or radiation therapy.

- **Genetic Counselor:** a specialist who will review your family history and other risk factors and advise you on how your relatives need to be evaluated.

- **Medical Oncologist:** a doctor who administers anti-cancer drugs or chemotherapy.

- **Pathologist:** a specialist who examines the tissue removed during a biopsy, and issues a report to help you and your doctor choose the most effective treatment.

- **Nurse Navigator:** a specially trained nurse who will be your guide during treatments, helping you overcome obstacles with education and support.

- **Nutritionist:** will advise you on what foods are best for your particular case and help you deal with complications from chemotherapy or surgery.

- **Personal Physician:** a surgeon, radiation oncologist, medical oncologist, or family physician who will be coordinating your treatment.

- **Physical Therapist:** a specialist who helps with post-surgical rehabilitation using exercise, heat, or massage.

- **Plastic Surgeon:** a surgeon with extensive additional training in cosmetic surgery, such as breast reconstruction after mastectomy.

- **Radiation Oncologist:** a physician trained in using high-energy X-rays for treatment.

- **Radiation Therapy Technologist:** works under the direction of the Radiation Oncologist to administer radiation treatment.

- **Social Worker:** will help you deal with social and economic aspects of treatment, such as helping find a support group or solving an insurance issue.

the same disease site (for example, breast or colon cancer patients), others by patient age or background. Some are just for patients; others include family or other special people.

Support groups give you a chance to openly discuss your thoughts with others who are going through the same experience. Many hospitals consider some form of group counseling to be part of the standard treatment—as necessary as an exercise class, for example.

Visit the support group a couple of times before joining, so you can be sure that the peer mix meets your needs and expectations.

GATHERING INFORMATION

When a woman hears that she has breast cancer, her first response may be a desire to have treatment—any treatment—immediately. But breast cancer is not a medical emergency like a heart attack or an appendicitis. By the time the tumor is found, it may have been growing for years. You can take several weeks to organize your thoughts, gather information, and make a decision about treatment, without jeopardizing the outcome.

Becoming well informed about breast cancer and about your options is one of the most important steps you can take at this stage. Knowledge of the facts will give you a sense of comfort and control.

Studies have shown that a woman's degree of satisfaction with the outcome of her treatment had to do less with the results of the treatment, and more with how much information she had when she made the decision. Take your time to gather all the facts you need, so that you can be comfortable with the decisions that will affect the rest of your life.

Your main source of information will be the professionals caring for you. Make lists of topics you want to discuss, and don't hesitate to ask any question, no matter how simple it may seem. Ask your support person to accompany you to the medical appointments, to help you take notes, tape record what was said, or ask additional questions.

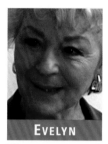

EVELYN

If you are not totally content with your physician, go and find somebody who will listen to you, answer your questions, and make you feel you are an important patient. A woman should be assertive and speak up, and if she wants to know why and when and where, she's entitled to these answers.

QUESTIONS TO ASK YOUR DOCTOR:

Could you give me the names of specialists you think I should see?

How about another set of names so I can choose the specialist(s) I like best?

Is there a multidisciplinary breast cancer team in the facility where you practice?

Tell me about your, or your colleagues' experience in dealing with breast cancer.

Both my husband and I are physicians. We thought we had at least mastered the vocabulary. But after listening to various options for an hour—radiation, brachytherapy, estrogen receptors, nipple reconstruction —we felt completely overwhelmed. It wasn't until the second or third visit that some of it started to make sense.

Many medical facilities have patient resource centers where you will find collections of books and DVDs on various aspects of breast cancer treatment.

On a regional or national level, there are several organizations that can be valuable sources of information. They can be found in the Resources section at the end of the book. The specialists at these organizations, many of whom are breast cancer survivors themselves, can answer many general questions about cancer, or send you written materials and information.

A lot of information—and, sadly, misinformation—is readily available on the internet. Be sure that the site you are consulting is sponsored by a reputable organization, and does not represent some individual's bias.

OVERVIEW OF TREATMENT OPTIONS

With today's early detection and improved treatment techniques, we can treat breast cancer more successfully than ever before.

The ultimate goal of any cancer treatment is to completely eliminate every single cancer cell from the body. This battle is usually waged on two fronts.

One line of attack uses *local treatments*: surgery and radiation therapy. Surgery removes the tumor. Radiation kills any cancer cells that might have been left in the breast area after the tumor was removed.

The other line of attack aims to destroy any cancer cells that might have broken away from the tumor, and traveled to distant parts of the body. This approach is called *systemic treatment*.

NINA-**Nurse Navigator**
If you find that the second opinion is completely different from the first, you may want to seek a third opinion. Beyond that, getting a fourth, fifth or sixth opinion delays treatment and creates confusion.

Systemic treatment can be in the form of chemotherapy (drugs that kill cancer cells), hormonal therapy (drugs that prevent cancer cells from growing), targeted therapy (drugs that help your body fight off cancer).

Don't worry if you feel confused by the new words and concepts presented here. Most people do at first. In the following days and weeks, as you explore this book, talk with your healthcare professionals, and gather additional information, you will begin to acquire the knowledge you need to make informed decisions.

Planning your treatment should involve your entire team of specialists, as well as your partner or your loved ones. Don't let anyone or anything make you feel rushed. With rare exceptions, breast cancer is not an emergency, and you can safely take several weeks to process the information.

GAYE

I kept a notebook right next to my bed—and whenever I would wake up with a burning question on my mind, I wrote it down. That way when I went to see the doctor, I was better prepared, and I didn't miss anything.

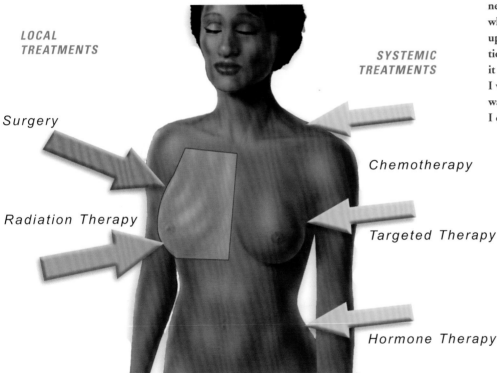

LOCAL TREATMENTS

SYSTEMIC TREATMENTS

Surgery

Chemotherapy

Radiation Therapy

Targeted Therapy

Hormone Therapy

The following chart of treatment options shows you how they might be used, alone or in combinations.

Almost always, you will begin with surgery: lumpectomy or mastectomy. If you have a lumpectomy, you will almost always have radiation therapy. If you have a mastectomy you might choose to have breast reconstruction. After either a lumpectomy or a mastectomy you might or might not have

CATHY

Know thy enemy. Know what you're facing and most of your fears will become manageable. That was the most important thing to me—to educate myself about breast cancer.

drug therapy (chemotherapy, hormone therapy or targeted therapy), depending on the characteristics of your tumor.

There are always exceptions. If your tumor is large, you may receive chemotherapy in order to shrink it before surgery. Past a certain age, it may not be beneficial to add radiation after a lumpectomy. Or you may have radiation treatment even if you had a mastectomy. These exceptions will be addressed in the appropriate chapters, and are best discussed with your treatment team.

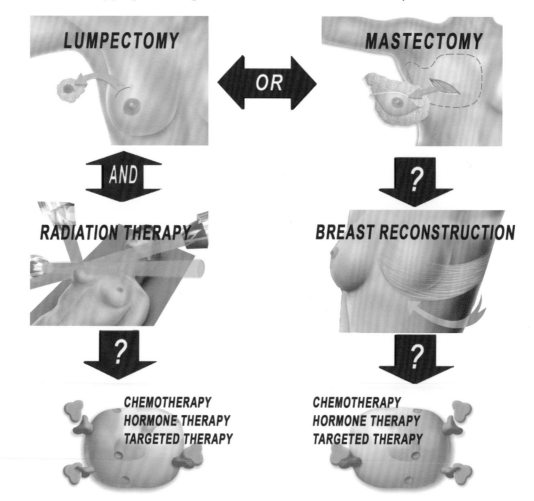

The key fact to remember is that it is *you* who will make the final decision, and all the members of the medical team need to respect it. That's why it is so important for you to learn all you can about your disease. The more information you can gather before you begin treatment, the more active the role you'll be able to take, and the better you will feel about your decision.

CHAPTER 2

BREAST CANCER BASICS

BREAST ANATOMY AND FUNCTION

First let's review the structure and function of the breast. Some of the terms like "lymph nodes" and "lobules" may be new to you, but they will help you understand breast cancer treatment better.

Although the general shape of a breast is circular or teardrop, breast tissue can be found from the collarbone to the bra line, and from the breastbone to the armpit. That is why it is important for you and your physician to examine that entire area during your breast examination.

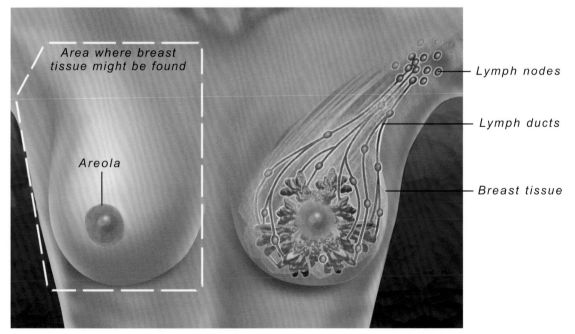

Anatomy of the breast area

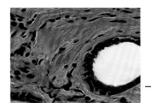

Duct, magnified x200

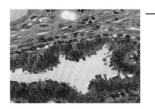

Lobe, magnified x200

lobe

duct

areola

Internal breast structures

Breasts are made up of milk-producing glands and milk-carrying ducts, imbedded in fatty tissue and fibrous supportive tissue. The glands are grouped in sections, called lobes. Each lobe has many smaller lobules that end in dozens of tiny grape-like bulbs where milk is produced. Slender tubes called ducts carry the milk from the lobes to the nipple. Most of the rest of the breast is composed of fatty tissue and fibrous supportive tissue.

Two muscles, the pectoralis major and the pectoralis minor, are attached to the ribs under the breast. One of these muscles may be cut to allow room for an implant. There are no muscles within the breast itself.

The area of darker skin around the nipple is called the areola.

Arteries and veins carry blood to and from the breast, supplying it with nutrients and oxygen.

An important concept to understand is the lymphatic system. Lymph is the fluid that leaks out of the blood vessels and accumulates between cells. Lymph ducts collect this fluid and return it to the main circulation. Along the way, lymphatic fluid is filtered through small bean-shaped structures called lymph nodes, which trap debris such as bacteria, or escaped cancer cells. You may think of the lymphatic system as a network of sewer lines.

Most of the lymphatic fluid from the breast drains toward the armpit area (the axilla), where it is filtered through the axillary lymph nodes. By examining these nodes, the surgeon can get a good indication of whether cancer cells have begun to escape from the breast toward the rest of the body.

How Breasts Grow and Change

From birth to old age, breasts go through more changes than almost any other organ in the body.

One to two years before menarche (first menstrual period) breasts begin to grow under the influence of the female hormones estrogen and progesterone.

During reproductive years, variations in the levels of these hormones cause the breasts to go through monthly cycles: milk glands become engorged and the breasts swell, as if getting ready for a pregnancy, then return to their inactive state again.

At menopause, levels of hormones drop, many milk producing glands shrink and disappear, and some of the breast tissue is replaced with fat.

All these changes sometimes damage the cells' DNA—the genetic material that tells the cell how to divide and grow. This damage may lead to cancer.

WHAT IS BREAST CANCER?

All organs in the body are made of cells. Individual cells are so small, they can be seen only through a microscope. Normally, cells divide in an orderly fashion to replace cells that have aged and died. Controls within each cell tell it to stop dividing if no new cells are needed.

Occasionally, damage to DNA during cell duplication may cause the controls to malfunction. Cells begin to divide uncontrollably, forming lumps or tumors.

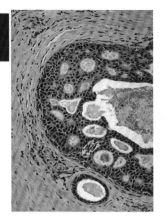

*Microscopic view
of cancer*

Tumors

The word "tumor" comes from a Latin word that means "swelling." A tumor could be composed of cells that divide excessively, but that do not invade or damage other parts of the body. A good example is a fibroid in the uterus, or a fibroadenoma in the breast. Both of these are called benign, that is, non-cancerous tumors.

Malignant tumors are composed of aggressively dividing cells that destroy surrounding tissues or travel to other parts of the body. In general conversation, the word "tumor" is often used to refer to a malignant condition, or cancer.

Growth Rate

Growth rate is the speed at which a lump or tumor grows. Different types of breast cancer grow at different rates. The time it takes for a tumor to become twice as large is called doubling time. The average doubling time for most breast cancer tumors is in the range of 50 to 200 days.

The change of the first normal cell into a malignant cell happens years before any evidence of cancer can be detected by any tests that we have today. It may take three to five years for a cluster of cancerous cells to become large enough to be seen on a mammogram. In other words, by the time your cancer has been detected, it has been there for several years. That is why there is no harm in taking a few more weeks to decide on the best treatment possible.

Risk Factors

Who is more likely to get breast cancer? All women are at risk for developing breast cancer. It is the most common cancer in women, with over 200,000 new cases being diagnosed every year. Breast cancer also occurs in men, but rarely.

The main predisposing factor—called risk factor—for breast cancer is age. The older you are, the greater your chances of developing the disease. Four out of five breast cancers are found in women over the age of fifty.

With a positive family history—having a first degree relative such as a mother, sister, or daughter who had breast cancer—a woman's risk of developing breast cancer increases. So women with breast cancer should suggest to their close female relatives that they consult their physicians about their own risk factors, and begin an effective program of early detection.

On the other hand, only about one in twenty cases of breast cancer is truly hereditary—that is, runs in the family—so not having a relative with breast cancer does not reduce the woman's risk.

Some of the other risk factors have a connection to the female hormone estrogen. Interruptions in the levels of this hormone, such as occur during pregnancy and lactation, seem to have a protective effect. In other words, fewer menstrual periods lead to a lower risk. That is probably why women who had one or more children by the age of thirty are at a lower risk, while women who had an early menarche (first menstrual period) or a late menopause (last period) are at a higher risk.

Age is the main risk factor for breast cancer

Recent studies indicate that use of certain forms of hormone replacement therapy, or HRT, popular for control of menopause symptoms, may increase a woman's chances of developing breast cancer. Use of low-dose birth control pills has not been linked to breast cancer.

Exercise and a low fat diet may have a protective effect, while alcohol intake of more than one drink per day may increase the risk.

While we don't know exactly what causes breast cancer, we do know that it is not caused by a blow or a physical injury and that it is definitely not contagious.

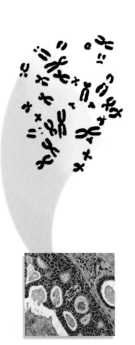

Cancer cells chromosomes contain genetic information errors

Breast Cancer Genes

An important step in understanding breast cancer has been the discovery of the genes that are linked to this disease—BRCA1 and BRCA2.

Genes are specific areas on chromosomes (strands of genetic material contained in our cells) that program the cell with information for growth and function. Scientists found that damage to specific genes on Chromosome 17 correlates with an increased incidence of hereditary-type breast cancer.

There are tests that can detect damage to the BRCA1 and BRCA2 gene. But widespread use of this test to identify women at high risk is being debated because the benefits and consequences of knowing the results are not clear. For example, a "negative" gene test does not mean that the gene is normal. Rather, it indicates that a mutation has not been found. A negative test does not guarantee that the woman will not get breast cancer. Today we can test for two genes, but many more will probably be discovered in the future.

Conversely, a "positive" test does not mean a woman will develop breast cancer, but it might open the door to a variety of problems if the woman's insurance company or employer were to obtain this information.

The best advice for a woman with breast cancer is to suggest to her relatives that they consult a qualified risk counselor before undergoing any genetic testing.

TYPES OF BREAST CANCER

Breast cancer types are named according to the part of the breast in which they develop. The most common forms of breast cancer come from cells that line the milk ducts (ductal cancer) or the milk-producing lobules (lobular cancer).

In the early stages, cancer cells divide locally, and do not cross the wall of the duct or lobule. This type of cancer is called *in situ*—meaning "in place." Once the cancer cells cross the lining of the duct or lobule, they are called *infiltrating*, or *invasive*. Do not be unduly alarmed if you are told your cancer is "invasive." Most cancers are, so your invasive cancer is the "normal" cancer.

Today about one in five cases of diagnosed breast cancers fall into the non-invasive, or in situ category—either *ductal carcinoma in situ* (DCIS), or *lobular carcinoma in situ* (LCIS).

DCIS cancers are highly curable. Some physicians don't even refer to them as cancer, but rather as "precancerous lesions," since DCIS may never progress to be an invasive cancer.

The treatment of DCIS, described in Chapter 11, may not follow the same plan as for invasive cancers, so we have dedicated a separate chapter to this non-invasive form of the disease. You still need to read the chapters on staging, surgery and radiation to understand the principles involved.

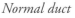
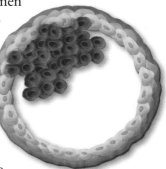

Normal duct

LCIS is a non-invasive growth that is not considered cancerous, but women who are diagnosed with LCIS have about a 1% per year risk of developing invasive breast cancer. That means that twenty years after diagnosis, the risk is about 18%. What is important to know is that the invasive cancer can occur in either breast, and not necessarily where the LCIS was originally found. In other words, LCIS is not a precursor, but a marker.

Infiltrating or invasive cancers, where malignant cells cross the lining of the duct or lobule, are more advanced than in situ cancers. They invade, or infiltrate, adjacent tissues. The most common type of breast cancer is the infiltrating ductal carcinoma. More than half of all cases are of this type.

In situ cancer

Other types of breast cancer are less common. One example is *Paget's Disease*, a cancerous growth that first appears as scaling on the nipple, and may be confused for a simple rash. Another is *inflammatory cancer*, a rare form of cancer that grows quickly, and causes redness and swelling of the breast. This is really the only form of breast cancer in which the treatment decision needs to be made as soon as possible.

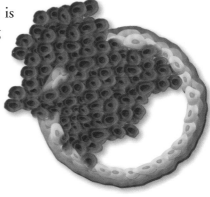

Invasive cancer

HOW CANCER SPREADS

As a malignant tumor grows, it may spread locally, invading and sometimes destroying other tissues, or cells may break away from the tumor and get into the lymphatic vessels, or into the blood vessels, and travel to distant parts of the body. Some of the breakaway cells will be trapped in the lymph nodes of the armpit, or axilla. Examination of these nodes by a procedure called axillary lymph node dissection, can help determine the stage (the degree of spread) of the cancer.

If cancer cells escape beyond the lymph nodes, or enter the circulatory system directly, they can spread to the liver, brain, lungs, and bones, forming new tumors called *metastases.* These distant metastases are the most worrisome, because they can damage vital organs. This advanced stage of breast cancer, called *metastatic* cancer, is less common and its management is more difficult.

To make sure that no cancer cells remain anywhere in the body, it is often necessary to use *systemic therapy*—therapy that reaches all the organs, in all parts of the body, by means of the blood stream. This is explained in the Chemotherapy, Hormone Therapy, and Targeted Therapy chapters.

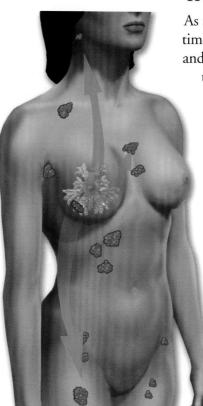

Cancer cells can metastasize to lung, bone, liver, and other organs

DIAGNOSIS AND STAGING

DIAGNOSIS

Biopsy

Mammography and ultrasound can detect "suspicious" lesions in the breast. But the only way to confirm a diagnosis of cancer is to perform a biopsy—that is, to remove a small piece of the tumor and have it examined under a microscope by a pathologist—a specialist in tumor identification.

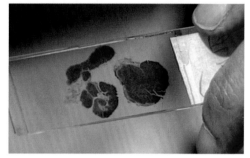

Tumor sample ready for examination under a microscope

Odds are that if you are reading this book, you already had a biopsy that showed that your tumor was malignant. If so, feel free to skip to the Staging section of this chapter.

Surgical Biopsy

The surgical biopsy is done under local anesthesia, sometimes with sedation. It takes about an hour, and causes minimal post-operative pain. And it does leave a small scar. The less invasive core biopsy is the first choice for most cases, but tumors close to the chest wall, or lack of suitable imaging equipment, may require a surgical approach.

Core Needle Biopsy

Today the *core needle biopsy* is considered be the standard of care because it provides reliable results without the need for a surgical procedure. It is done under a local anesthetic and takes only a few minutes.

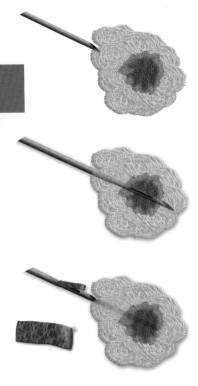

Core needle taking
a biopsy sample

The core biopsy is performed with a device that works like an ear-piercing instrument: it propels a large needle very rapidly through the lesion. A special notch in the needle traps a sliver of tissue for examination. Samples obtained with core biopsy are large enough to be cut into thin slices for better examination under the microscope.

TUMOR TESTING

After the biopsy, the sample of tumor will be examined under a microscope by a pathologist, who will identify the cells and determine whether the tumor is benign or malignant. If the tumor is malignant, many additional tests will be carried out in order to select the most effective treatment.

Invasive or in situ

It is important to determine whether the cancer cells are growing within the lobules or ducts (in situ) or have begun to penetrate the lining and invade the surrounding breast tissue (invasive). The treatment for an in situ cancer will be different from the one for the more serious invasive cancer.

Hormone Receptor Status

A *receptor* is an area on the surface of a cell that can bind with specific substances, much like a lock accepts a key.

Tumors that have estrogen or progesterone receptors are called estrogen receptor (ER) positive, or progesterone receptor (PR) positive, or hormone receptor positive (HR). In these tumors, when the hormone binds to its receptor, it activates the cell, making it divide, and helping the tumor grow.

This information is important, because hormone receptor positive tumors can be treated with drugs that block the action of hormones. Tumors lacking hormone receptors are less likely to respond to hormone therapy.

HER2/neu

Women with an abnormally high level of a substance called HER2/neu tend to develop much more aggressive breast cancers. A test will determine your level of HER2/neu and help your oncologist decide if you are a good candidate for treatment with drugs such as Herceptin.

What is a Triple-Negative Breast Cancer?

Having a triple-negative breast cancer means your tumor tested "negative" for estrogen receptors (ER-), progesterone receptors (PR-), and HER2. This cancer does not respond to hormonal therapy (such as tamoxifen or aromatase inhibitors) or therapies that target HER2 receptors, such as Herceptin. Other medicines will need to be used. More than one out of every ten women are found to be triple-negative.

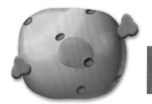

Estrogen binding to receptor sites

Cell Grade

The appearance of your tumor cells is an indication of how aggressive the cancer is. Cells that look almost normal may be scored as Grade 1. If they are moderately deformed they may be Grade 2. And if their shape is bizarre and differs a lot from normal cells, they are called Grade 3. Grade 1 cancers may be easier to treat.

> *My tumor is a ...*
> *It is hormone receptor ...*
> *and HER2 ...*

GENOMIC TESTING

Each person's cancer has a unique combination of genetic changes. Analyzing the tumor to identify these changes is called DNA sequencing, or genetic or genomic testing. Newly developed tests called genomic testing can evaluate a large number of genes in a tumor tissue sample. This information can be very valuable in deciding whether a particular tumor will respond to a specific treatment.

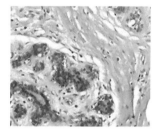

Normal breast cells

In certain cases, these gene assays can measure the likelihood of distant breast cancer recurrence, and help your healthcare team decide if chemotherapy should be recommended in a particular case.

Oncotype DX is a genomic test that analyzes the activity of a group of genes that can affect how a cancer is likely to behave. It is both a prognostic test, since it provides more information about how likely (or unlikely) the breast cancer is to come back, and a predictive test, since it predicts the likelihood of benefit from chemotherapy or radiation therapy treatment.

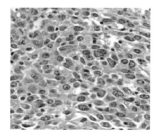

High grade breast cancer

The results can help your healthcare team predict your chances that the cancer might come back, and identify the most effective therapies for successful treatment. Ask your health care provider to discuss the possibility of tumor DNA sequencing as part of your care.

Personalized Medicine

Cancer specialists are now using these gene-based diagnostic tests in various ways to plan more effective treatments. Tests that analyze dozens of genes in the tumor to help women and their doctors make decisions about whether or not to include chemotherapy in their treatment plan, or whether the cancer has a low or high risk of recurrence within ten years after diagnosis.

Genomic testing is rapidly becoming the foundation and the gold standard of "personalized medicine".

THE PATHOLOGY REPORT

Your treatment will be based on the precise identification of the cells in your tumor. To be absolutely sure, the biopsy is often examined by two or more pathologists. Their report, although still preliminary, will generally take several days. Many women find waiting to be very distressing.

The *final report* can only be issued after the tumor and the lymph nodes are removed during surgery. This report will specify the size of the tumor, the type of cell the tumor is composed of, and whether there is tumor spread to lymph nodes. This information is essential for planning your treatment.

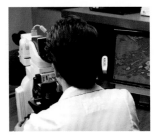

ADDITIONAL TESTS

Why more tests? A biopsy can confirm that the diagnosis is cancer, but it will not show whether the cancer has spread to other parts of the body. This information is important to determine the stage of the tumor.

Therefore, additional tests may be needed, including blood tests, CAT scans or MRIs of the abdomen or other parts of the body, and bone scans.

MRI

MRI or Magnetic Resonance Imaging uses a combination of magnetic energy and ordinary radio waves to create images of the inside of your body.

You may have an MRI scan of both your breasts. This MRI will give the surgeon a more accurate idea of the size, shape and location of any additional tumors that may be present in either breast.

A body MRI will look for possible distant spread of the cancer. Because the MRI unit can feel cramped, notify the technologist or your physician if you feel uncomfortable in confined spaces. An MRI is painless, and does not expose you to X-ray radiation. The test takes about an hour.

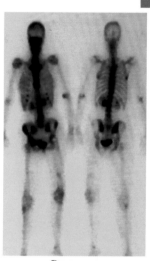

Bone scan

Bone Scan

Some of the more common sites to which breast cancer cells may metastasize, or spread, include bones. The most effective way to find these metastases is to perform a nuclear scan. This test is generally done if the tumor is large, or the lymph nodes are positive and there is a good chance that tumor cells may be found in other areas of the body.

For this scan, tiny amounts of radioactive substance are injected into a vein. Once inside the body, the radioactive substance concentrates in areas where there is an unusually increased number of blood vessels—a "hot spot"—that may correspond to a new growth of cancer cells.

CT Scan

CAT scan, CT scan, or Computerized Axial Tomography all mean the same thing. This test uses ordinary X-rays, and a rotating film/source system to obtain detailed images of your body. The test is short and painless.

PET/CT Scan

The PET scan works on a principle similar to the bone scan. One of the newest and most valuable imaging techniques is the combination of PET scans, which reflect tissue function, with CT scans, which show tissue structure. This combination provides outstanding information for diagnosis and treatment of cancer.

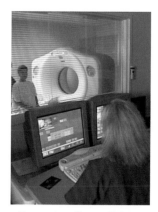

Preparing for a CT scan

STAGING

Why Staging?

Each cancer is unique, each woman is different, and the combination of treatment options is practically endless. To help determine who should get what treatment, cancer specialists rely on *staging*—a system that places the cancer into a certain group. The stage of your tumor is the most important factor in deciding what treatment is best for you.

TNM

In simplified form, staging is based on: the size of the tumor; presence of cancer cells in the lymph nodes; and metastasis, or spread, to other organs. This is the so-called TNM—tumor, node, metastasis—staging system.

Tumor size is determined when the tumor is removed and sent to the pathologist.

Lymph nodes are checked for evidence of tumor spread at the time of surgery in a procedure called axillary lymph node dissection.

Metastasis, or spread to other organs, is assessed with bone scans, CT scans, and blood tests.

Putting all this information together is called *staging*.

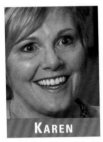

KAREN

Early on I decided I wasn't going to let my head wander. You can imagine all sort of scenarios and most of them aren't true.

The stage of MY tumor is.....

STAGES OF BREAST CANCER

Stage 0 (in situ)

Non-invasive breast cancer (DCIS, LCIS). No cancer cells have penetrated the lining of the duct or lobule.

Stage I

Invasive tumor, 2 cm (3/4 inch) or smaller. Axillary lymph nodes are negative and there is no evidence of distant metastases.

Stage II

Tumor is 2-5 cm in size (about 3/4 to 2 inches). Axillary lymph nodes may or may not be positive for cancer. Even if the tumor is smaller than 2 cm, but the lymph nodes are positive, cancer is also considered Stage II.

Stage III

Tumor is larger than 5 cm (2 inches) with extensive lymph node spread. Tumor may extend into the pectoral muscles or into the skin of the breast, but there are no distant metastases.

Stage IV

If the tumor has spread to other organs, usually lungs, liver, bone and brain, it is Stage IV regardless of its size, or of the number of positive axillary lymph nodes.

Ask your doctor to draw the size of YOUR tumor.

*TUMORS,
ACTUAL SIZE*

1 cm

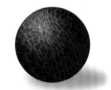

2 cm

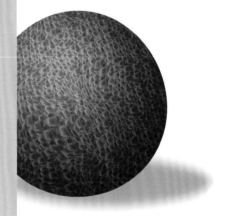

5 cm

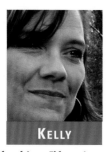

KELLY

One of the things I'd say is, "Don't rush to make a decision. Don't let anybody rush you." There is a lot of information to gather, and to absorb, and to see what applies to you. If you rush now, you might regret it later.

KAREN

You are suddenly presented with an array of options. It is overwhelming. Am I supposed to do a mastectomy? Or a lumpectomy? Yes or no on the reconstruction? It is a very personal decision. What does your breast mean to you? What is your self image?

Treatment Options

You may find it helpful to think of stage as degree of risk presented by a particular tumor.

At one end of the scale are the low-risk situations: very tiny tumors that have not spread to lymph nodes, and that are composed of cells that are not very aggressive.

Further along are slightly larger tumors, still smaller than about a half inch (1 cm), still without evidence of lymph node spread, but often more aggressive.

At the other end of the scale are the situations that involve the greatest risk: larger tumors that have invaded the lymph nodes.

If you are at the low-risk end of the scale, your treatment may require breast conserving surgical removal of the tumor plus a course of radiation therapy, for certain age groups, and perhaps a less aggressive form of hormonal therapy or chemotherapy.

Larger tumors may be treated with more aggressive chemotherapy, sometimes starting it before surgery (neo-adjuvant chemotherapy).

For high-risk tumors, at the far end of the scale, there are a wide variety of options, including dose-dense chemotherapy.

CHAPTER 4

SURGERY

To ensure the best chance for success, it is important to remove all the cancerous tissue from the breast and from the rest of the body. The first step is usually surgery to remove the tumor from the breast area, sometimes combined with radiation therapy. Chemotherapy might be added to deal with any cancer cells that might have left the breast area and spread to other parts.

Over the past 50 years the trend in breast cancer surgery has been to achieve the best cancer control possible, while removing less and less normal breast tissue. Studies have shown that removing more tissue does not lower the chance of cancer recurrence in the area.

Today, *oncoplastic surgery* is rapidly becoming the standard of care of surgical treatement. Oncoplastic surgery combines cancer control, with the most pleasing cosmetic results possible, including a symmetric appearance.

Breast Surgery Options

There are two surgical options: One is to remove just the tumor, with a safety margin of healthy breast tissue around it, conserving most of the breast. This is called wide local excision, partial mastectomy, or *lumpectomy*. This *breast-conserving* surgery is commonly followed by radiation therapy—treatment of the breast area with high energy X-rays to destroy any cancer cells that may have remained behind. The combined approach is called *breast conserving therapy*, or BCT.

The other option is to remove the entire breast in a procedure called *mastectomy*. There are many mastectomy techniques used today. They will be described in the next chapter.

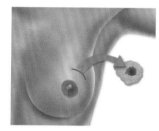

Lumpectomy: removal of the tumor with a safety margin of healthy tissue.

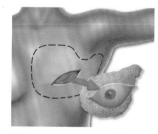

Mastectomy: removal of the entire breast.

LUMPECTOMY

What is a Lumpectomy?

If the tumor is small, you may have the option of having **breast-conserving surgery**. The goal of this procedure is to remove the whole tumor, while conserving as much breast tissue as possible. A margin of normal tissue is also removed to make sure no malignant cells are left behind.

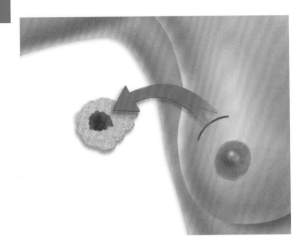

The technical term for this type of surgery is *partial mastectomy*. Most people commonly refer to it as a *lumpectomy*—a "lump-removal", so to speak. Depending on how much breast tissue is removed, the procedure may be called *wide excision, segmental mastectomy*, or *quadrantectomy*. The specific technique may vary from surgeon to surgeon and from case to case.

An **oncoplastic surgeon** will be able to choose the best approach for your cancer operation based on the size of your breasts, the location of the tumor, and the amount of droop in your breasts.

Your surgeon may recommend pre-treating the tumor with chemotherapy in order to shrink it before surgery. This reduces the amount of tissue that needs to be removed during surgery. This is called *neoadjuvant* chemotherapy.

The cosmetic result of breast conserving surgery will vary with the location and size of the tumor, and the size of the breast. Removing a large tumor from a large breast may result in a normal-looking breast, but removing even a small tumor from a small breast may lead to noticeable change in breast size and shape that may be cosmetically unacceptable.

Today's advances in oncoplastic surgery make it possible to combine the removal of the tumor with a larger but better-shaped volume of breast tissue. With a simple breast reduction on the other side, it is possible to achieve both tumor control and very pleasing cosmetic results.

Breast conserving surgery usually requires additional treatment of the breast area with high energy X-rays (*radiation therapy*) to kill any surviving cancer cells that might be left behind. This combination is called **breast conserving treatment**, or BCT.

QUESTIONS TO ASK YOUR SURGEON:

Is lumpectomy an option for me? Why or why not?

How will my breast look after the treatment? Can you show me pictures?

How much pain should I expect in the first few days?

How long before I can go back to my regular activities?

Before Surgery

If you are being treated by a specialist for an underlying condition, you will need pre-operative clearance. Be sure to schedule it well before your surgery.

A lumpectomy may be done in a hospital or in an outpatient surgery center. Have a friend or relative accompany you to the hospital, to meet you after surgery and to drive you home if you are discharged the same day.

If your tumor is difficult to feel, your surgeon will have a *localization procedure* done before you go to surgery. An ultrasound probe or a special mammography unit will be used to pinpoint the location of the tumor and insert a thin wire directly into it, so the surgeon can find the tumor during surgery.

Another way is to place a tiny radioactive seed or a magnetic marker into the tumor, and use it as a homing beacon during the procedure. The advantage is that these can be placed days or weeks before the procedure, greatly reducing the workload on the morning of surgery.

If you are having oncoplastic surgery, your surgeon will meet you in the pre-op area to draw markings on your skin where the incisions will be made to achieve the best result possible.

You'll speak with the anesthesiologist to decide whether you'll have general or local anesthesia, depending on your health and personal preferences.

You'll also be asked to sign an informed consent form as an indication that you understand the procedure and the possible complications, such as infection and bleeding. Make sure to read the form carefully and ask for explanations of any parts that you are not comfortable with.

If you are having a *sentinel lymph node biopsy procedure* (described later in this chapter) at the time of the lumpectomy, the surgeon will inject a small amount of a special substance into the breast area to highlight the sentinel node later during surgery.

Just before you go into the operating room a nurse will start an intravenous line and give you something to help you relax.

QUESTIONS TO ASK YOUR ANESTHESIOLOGIST:

What will I feel and hear if I have local anesthesia?

Will you give me something to control the pain after I wake up from the anesthetic?

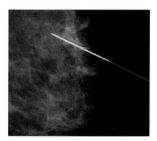

Breast needle localization X-ray

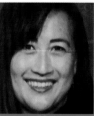

NINA-Nurse Navigator

Sometime before surgery, talk with your anesthesiologist to address any concerns you may have about nausea, pain or anxiety. She or he will have ways to relieve your symptoms.

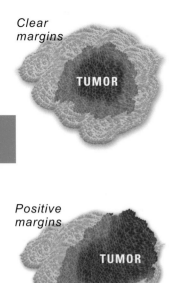

Clear margins

Positive margins

The Surgical Procedure

A lumpectomy takes less than an hour. The surgeon will remove the tumor with a margin of surrounding healthy breast tissue. This margin, about one-half to three-quarters of an inch in thickness, helps decrease the chance that tumor cells are left behind.

The surgical specimen will be sent to a pathologist who will examine it under a microscope and make a **preliminary** assessment of whether the *margins are clear* of tumor cells. If tumor cells are found along the edges, it means that some cancerous cells may have been left behind, and more tissue needs to be removed while you are still in the operating room.

The **final** assessment takes two-to-four days to complete, because the pathologist needs time to stain the edges of the tissue in order to see the different cells better. If cancerous cells are found around the margins at that time, you may need to return for a repeat lumpectomy.

The surgeon will place several metal clips in the lumpectomy cavity to show the radiation concologist where the tumor was, and to help interpret future mammograms.

The surgeon may also place a plastic tube called a *drain* to collect any fluid that may accumulate in the surgical area. This drain will be removed when it no longer drains fluid, usually within a few days.

By using oncoplastic procedures, the surgeon will be able to achieve effective cancer control together with a pleasing cosmetic result. Often a procedure on the other breast will restore the symmetric look. Be sure to get detailed information before the procedure as to what is possible in your case.

Recovery After Lumpectomy

After the lumpectomy, you'll be taken to the recovery room for a short while. Depending on the procedure you had, you may be discharged to go home. In general, you will be able to resume normal activities soon after surgery.

Have your pain medication prescription filled before you go home. Take the pills as necessary, instead of "powering through" the pain. Effective pain management improves your quality of life and helps promote healing.

NINA-Nurse Navigator

You will learn how to empty the drain and measure the output before going home. Write down the amount each time as instructed and show it to your physician at the post-op appointment.

If you're going home with a drain inserted, you'll need to empty the fluid from the detachable drain bulb a few times a day. Make sure you understand the instructions on caring for the drain before you leave the hospital.

Take sponge baths instead of showers until your drains and any staples or sutures have been removed.

Be diligent about doing whatever exercise routine you are assigned after surgery to prevent arm and shoulder stiffness.

Watch for signs of infection in your incision and call the surgeon's office if any of them appear.

Wear a supportive bra day and night for a while to minimize any movement that could cause pain. Women with larger breasts may find it more comfortable to sleep on the side that has not been operated on, with the healing breast supported by a pillow.

Weeks or months after surgery, as the damaged nerves regrow, you may feel itching or shooting pains, and you may be very sensitive to touch. This sensation may last for months or years, but the frequency may decrease in time.

Radiation Therapy

An important part of breast conserving treatment is radiation therapy. Radiation therapy uses high energy X-rays applied to the breast area to kill any remaining cancer cells. You can learn more about the different options for radiation therapy in Chapter 6.

Is Lumpectomy Right for Me?

Should you have a lumpectomy with radiation, or a mastectomy? Research involving thousands of women and many years of follow-up, shows that there is **no difference in survival** between the two approaches. Despite these very conclusive studies, some physicians may still favor mastectomy over breast conserving surgery. This may be due to personal bias, or to reliance on information that is now obsolete, or for very valid medical reasons.

If your doctor does not offer you a lumpectomy as an option, make sure you understand why.

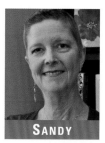

SANDY

My tumor was small and my breasts are large, so having a lumpectomy left very little change. And I read enough to know that lumpectomy is as good as a mastectomy in terms of getting rid of the cancer. I am comfortable with my decision.

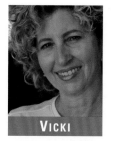

VICKI

I had a lumpectomy. It was extremely easy and when it was over I felt physically very good. I was able to go home with relatively little pain.

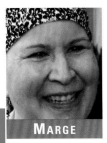

MARGE

The surgeon said, "I'll use oncoplastic procedures to reconstruct your breast, and do a little breast lift on the other side to make them even." And the next day I looked down, and "Oh my, these don't look like they nursed five children."

QUESTIONS TO ASK:

How much pain should I expect after the procedure?

Do I need to arrange to have someone help me with daily activities?

How long before I can go back to my work?

Besides being equally effective, breast conserving surgery offers several advantages over a mastectomy. You keep your breast, (although you may notice a change in shape), and you avoid the emotional trauma of losing the breast. A good cosmetic result can be expected. Unless the tumor was close to the nipple, nipple sensation can usually be preserved, although for a time the nipple sensation may be painful rather than pleasurable.

Not all women can have breast conserving surgery. You need to meet certain criteria, or a lumpectomy will not be recommended.

**Usually (but not always)
a lumpectomy would not be recommended if:**

• The tumor is so big or the breast so small that the cosmetic result would not be satisfactory after removal of the tumor.
• The tumor involves the skin.
• You are not willing to have radiation therapy, or there is no convenient radiation therapy facility near you.
• You already had one course of radiation to that breast.
• You have connective tissue disease such as lupus or vasculitis.
• You want to have a mastectomy as a personal preference.

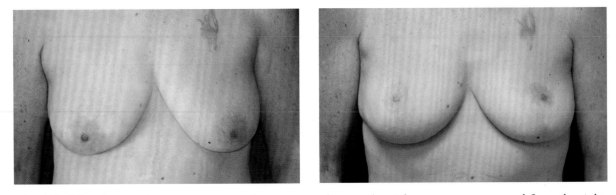

In skilled hands, oncoplastic surgery can achieve outstanding results. The tumor was removed from the right breast (left photo). A "breast lift" was done on the left breast to achieve a symmetrical look.
Photos courtesy Juliann Reiland, MD

MASTECTOMY

What is a Mastectomy?

Mastectomy, or surgical removal of the breast, has been used to treat breast cancer for several centuries.

The early *radical mastectomy*, which removed the entire breast, the lymph nodes in the armpit, and one of the major muscles of the chest wall, was based on the mistaken belief that the more tissue removed, the better the chances of curing the cancer. Today it is rarely used, and only for very extensive cancers that spread to the muscles.

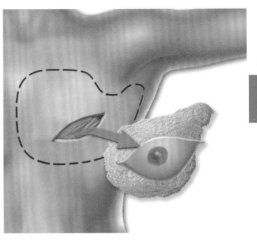

In a conventional mastectomy the nipple, areola and some skin are removed

In the 1970s and 1980s, research proved that there was no advantage in removing the chest muscles. This led to the *modified radical mastectomy*, a procedure that removes as much of the breast tissue as possible, including the nipple and the areola, and a number of axillary lymph nodes, but not the muscles.

Multiple options for mastectomy are available today:

The *simple mastectomy*, with or without reconstruction.

The *skin-sparing mastectomy* that preserves most of the breast skin envelope. Many women choose to have it because it leaves a natural skin pouch that makes it easier to have an immediate reconstruction, either with implants or with your own tissues, and it yields some of the most realistic and pleasing results.

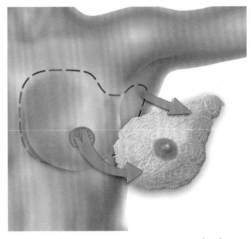

In a skin-sparing mastectomy only the nipple and areola are removed

The *nipple-sparing mastectomy* preserves the entire skin envelope and the nipple and areola. However the woman loses sensation in the nipple 95% of the time.

A skin-sparing or a nipple-sparing mastectomy is not right for you if you have decided against immediate reconstruction, or if the tumor is too close to the skin.

QUESTIONS TO ASK YOUR
ANESTHESIOLOGIST:

Will you give me something
to help me relax before
surgery?

How long will it take me to
get back to normal after
a general anesthetic?

What are the side effects of
anesthesia?

THINGS TO TAKE WITH
YOU TO THE HOSPITAL:

- reading glasses
- nightgown
- slippers
- toiletries
- something to read
- favorite pillow
- cell phone and charger
- change of loose
  clothing for going home

NINA-Nurse Navigator

Don't be annoyed because
every staff person seems
to ask you for your full
name and birthdate, over
and over. It is done to
make sure you get the
right procedure.

Before Surgery

A mastectomy is usually done in a hospital under general anesthesia. After a date is set, someone on your surgeon's staff will review with you the admission process for the particular hospital where the operation will take place. Find out whether your insurance covers surgical fees, hospital room, anesthesiologist's fees, and other charges.

If applicable, obtain a medical clearance from whatever specialists may be treating you for other medical conditions, and make sure the necessary paperwork was sent to your surgeon well in advance.

List all the medications you are taking, both prescription and over-the-counter, since some of them may have adverse effects during anesthesia or surgery. (For example, aspirin-containing preparations can increase bleeding.) Be sure to mention allergies, smoking history, colds or tooth decay.

Blood transfusions are rarely needed during lumpectomies or mastectomies, but may be required for certain types of breast reconstruction. Ask your physician about donating and storing your own blood before your surgery so that it can be used, should you need it.

Pack all the personal belongings you may need: a nightgown, slippers, toiletries, books or perhaps a favorite pillow, and a change of loose clothing that buttons in front, to wear when you go home.

Most people undergoing surgery enjoy having a friend or relative accompany them to the hospital and meet them after the procedure. If you are going to be sent home the same day, you will definitely need someone to drive you.

You'll be instructed not to eat or drink anything after midnight on the night before the surgery.

On the day of the surgery, you'll first go through an admission process at the hospital. The hospital staff will ask you to sign an informed consent form listing your doctor's name and the name of the surgical procedure you are having. Make sure you feel comfortable with what you are signing. If there is anything on the form that worries you, ask to see your doctor.

Your surgeon will meet you in the pre-op area to draw markings on your skin where the incisions will be made to achieve the best result possible.

The Surgical Procedure

An intravenous line (an "IV") will be started in one of your arms, and you may get something to help you relax.

When the surgical team is ready, you will be taken to the operating room. Several devices will be attached to you, such as an automatic blood pressure cuff, a heart monitor, and a blood oxygen monitor. The anesthesiologist will inject a drug into your vein through the tubing, and you will fall asleep almost immediately. A breathing device may be placed through your mouth to maintain a way for you to breathe during the surgery. Your blood pressure, pulse, and breathing will be monitored during the entire procedure.

The mastectomy procedure can take up to two to three hours. Breast tissue extends from the collar bone to the edge of the ribs, and from the breast bone to the muscles in the back of the armpit, and all of it needs to be removed.

The tissue will be sent to the pathologist, who will examine it for evidence of cancer spread beyond the breast. Preliminary results may be available while you are still in the operating room. Final results may take weeks.

You may also undergo a procedure called an axillary lymph node dissection. It is described later in this chapter.

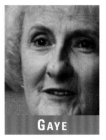

GAYE

I was not happy about having to deal with drains. The nurse showed me how to use them, and I said, "I don't think I can do this." But I did, and my husband helped.

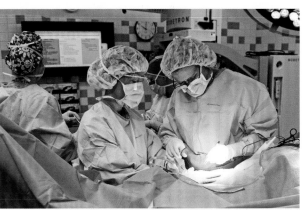

Surgeons performing a mastectomy
Photo courtesy Avera Breast Center

When your surgery is completed, one or two tubes called drains will be placed under the skin to help remove the fluid that accumulates at the site of surgery. Before you go home, you'll be shown how to empty the suction bulbs attached to the drains and how to keep a record of the volume and color of the fluid. The drains will be removed at a follow-up visit to your surgeon, or as soon as the drainage decreases to less than about an ounce.

If you've decided to have immediate reconstruction of the breast, the plastic surgeon will take over while you are still asleep.
Reconstruction can be done using your own tissues or using a synthetic implant. The procedure may take anywhere from an hour to six or eight hours, depending on the method used. You can learn about reconstruction in more detail in Chapter 5.

Recovery After Mastectomy

After surgery, you'll be taken to the recovery room. As you wake up from the anesthetic, you may feel cold, and your throat may be sore from the tube used for anesthesia. You may fade between waking and sleeping for several hours.

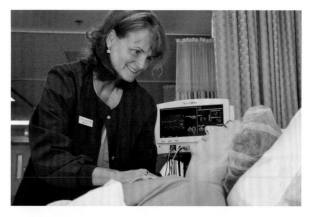

After surgery, you will be taken to the recovery room

Whatever surgery they are going to have, most women like to have a friend or relative meet them after the operation. You can ask your surgeon how long it will take before you will be brought to your room after surgery and to arrange with the hospital to allow that person to meet you there.

Most women will stay in the hospital for one or two nights after a mastectomy, and somewhat longer after a mastectomy with reconstruction.

Each woman reacts to surgery differently. Most can take a short walk in and out of their hospital room the day of surgery. The next day, most are able to eat a regular diet and get around.

Recovering at Home

Once you're home, you'll probably feel more tired than usual for a while. Don't be discouraged. You've just been through general anesthesia and major surgery, and fatigue is to be expected.

Take sponge baths for a few days after surgery and don't shower until your drains are removed, and the surgeon tells you that it is alright to get the incision wet. When you do shower, treat the skin gently and pat, rather than rub, the incision.

Immediately after surgery, you'll probably have trouble moving your arm due to muscle tightness and soreness around the shoulder. Use the arm as tolerated immediately after surgery, but avoid active stretching or pulling until the drains are removed and you get your doctor's approval. Don't be afraid to enlist the help of a friend or relative until your arm function returns.

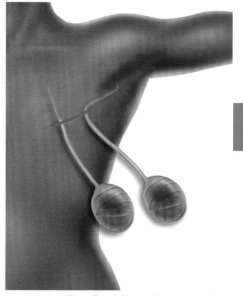

Drains collect fluid from the surgical site

Many women return to work as soon as they feel better, even while their chemotherapy and radiation treatments are continuing. If your job requires lifting or strenuous physical activity, you may need to change your activities until you have fully regained your strength.

Risks of Mastectomy

Like all surgeries, mastectomy has some risks. You may experience numbness in the upper inner arm and armpit area, caused by injury to one of the nerves. If this happens to you, you may need to be particularly careful when you shave your underarm. The numbness will usually improve over months or years, but the sensation may never be completely normal.

You may develop a fluid collection under the scar that may need to be drained with a needle by your physician.

Wound healing problems or wound infections may also occur, although rarely. A side effect of axillary lymph node dissection is swelling of the arm, called lymphedema. This is described later in this chapter.

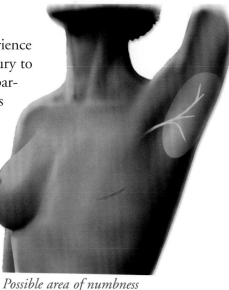

Possible area of numbness after surgery

49

Exercises After Mastectomy

The goal of exercising your shoulder and arm after surgery is to regain the full range of motion as soon as possible. But don't attempt to begin exercising without specific instructions from your healthcare provider.

Exercises must be done in stages. After the drains are removed, your doctor or physical therapist may assign pendulum-like movements with your arm, to begin loosening any tightness in the shoulder area.

• Holding on to something for support (such as a chair or desk), lean forward at the waist and swing your arm in gradually enlarging circles. Make ten circles, rest, then repeat in the other direction.

After the sutures are removed, you may be told to begin stretching exercises to regain full motion in the shoulder.

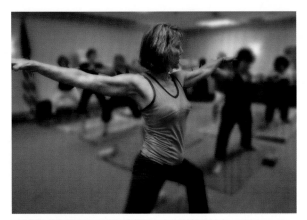

Yoga offers both physical and mental benefits

• Walk your fingers up the wall, until you feel mild pain in the incision, and note how far you can reach each day.

• Throw a rope or an old tie over a door, and move your arms up and down in a see-saw motion.

• Walk your arm up your back as far as you can.

Many communities and some medical centers offer swimming, exercise, based fitness programs and dance classes specifically for breast cancer patients.

Is Mastectomy Right for Me?

Numerous research studies, involving thousands of women and many years of follow-up, show that there is no difference in **survival** in patients treated with lumpectomy and radiation, or with mastectomy.

There is a slightly higher rate of **local** cancer recurrence (in the breast area itself) following lumpectomy. One out of a hundred women treated with lumpectomy will develop a local recurrence within a year. (In other words, there is a 1% per year recurrence rate. The chance of having a recurrence within ten years is 10%.) Local recurrences are not life threatening, and can be controlled by performing a mastectomy at the time that the cancer recurrence is found. Since there is no difference in numbers of life-threatening distant metastases (cancer in other sites of the body) between lumpectomy and mastectomy, there is no difference in life expectancy between the two procedures.

So the choice is between running a slightly higher risk of a local recurrence (which is not life threatening) following lumpectomy, or accepting a mastectomy.

The **advantages** of a mastectomy are that usually no radiation therapy is required (unless your lymph nodes had cancer cells in them, or the tumor was very near the chest wall), and there is a decreased risk of local recurrence. Some women prefer the mastectomy because of the peace of mind they expect after the removal of the entire cancerous breast.

The **disadvantages** of mastectomy include the need for more extensive surgery, and the emotional impact of losing the entire breast, probably including the nipple.

Your choice will be dictated by various factors. It is important to remember that no decision needs to be made overnight. You can take up to several weeks to gather information. You do not need to make the decision alone. Consult your healthcare professionals, get a second opinion, and talk with your loved ones. Ask your nurse navigator or your surgeon how you can connect with other women who had the procedure so you can find out about their experience.

Lumpectomy or Mastectomy?

Many women do not realize that they can choose between lumpectomy and mastectomy without compromising their life expectancy, or their chance of distant metastases. **Studies have proven that breast-conserving therapy (lumpectomy plus radiation therapy) is as effective as a mastectomy.** In other words, *survival* from breast cancer is the same whether you have mastectomy or lumpectomy with radiation. Removing your breasts will not guarantee you will live longer.

Review the pros and cons of each procedure. Then, in consultation with your healthcare team, and armed with an open mind, you can pick the procedure that you feel is best for you.

ADVANTAGES OF MASTECTOMY:

- usually no radiation therapy required, unless
    lymph nodes are involved
        the cancer is too close to the skin
        the cancer is larger than 5 cm
- important for some women's peace of mind
        but does not stop cancer that spread,
        so peace of mind is false

ADVANTAGES OF LUMPECTOMY:

- breast is spared
- preserves nipple and skin sensation
- yields good cosmetic results

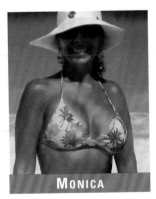

MONICA

I had a mastectomy with reconstruction. But you should see the attention I get at the beach!

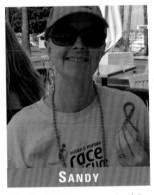

SANDY

I had a lumpectomy. And I am completely confident in my decision.

Questions to consider when making your choice between mastectomy and lumpectomy:

- Is the appearance of my breast after surgery important to me?

- If it isn't now, how might I feel in one year? In ten years?

- Is my surgical team skilled in oncoplastic surgery?

- Is the sensitivity in my breast after surgery important to me?

- If I have breast-conserving surgery, do I need, and am I willing, to have a course of radiation therapy?

- If I want radiation therapy, am I able to travel to the facility five days a week for five-to-seven weeks for treatments?

- If not, does my surgeon offer other options that are of shorter duration, like five days of brachytherapy?

- Is intraoperative radiation therapy possible or advisable for me?

- If I have a mastectomy, do I also want breast reconstruction surgery? And surgery on the other side for symmetry?

- What treatment does my insurance cover, and what do I have to pay for?

Write down the pros and cons of lumpectomy and mastectomy the way YOU see them.

QUESTIONS TO ASK YOUR DOCTOR:

Is lumpectomy an option for me? Why or why not?

Does a mastectomy decrease the chances of the cancer coming back?

How will I look after a mastectomy if I decide against reconstruction?

Can you show me pictures?

Can you refer me to a plastic surgeon so I can discuss my reconstruction options?

What kind of reconstruction procedure do you think would be best for me?

Who can I talk to about my concerns about appearance, dating, pregnancy, etc?

AXILLARY LYMPH NODE DISSECTION

Whether you've had a mastectomy or a lumpectomy for invasive cancer, you may also have a procedure called *axillary lymph node dissection*: some of the lymph nodes from your armpit will be removed and examined for evidence of cancer spread. This information is extremely important for deciding whether you will need additional therapy.

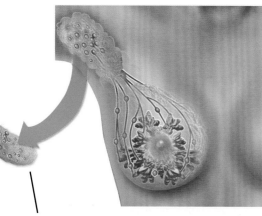

Axillary lymph nodes and fat are removed for examination

What exactly are *lymph nodes?* Arteries, veins and capillaries carry blood to and from various parts of the body. Some fluid, called *lymph* seeps out of these blood vessels, and is returned to the blood stream by a network of thin tubes called *lymphatic ducts*.

The lymph is filtered through tiny bean-shaped organs called *lymph nodes*. Foreign particles (such as bacteria from an infection in the finger, or break-away cancer cells from a tumor in the breast) are trapped in the lymph nodes before they can enter the general circulation. Lymph from the breast area usually drains through lymph nodes located in the armpit, also called the axilla.

For an axillary lymph node dissection the surgeon will remove a portion of the fat pad from the armpit, with ten to twenty imbedded lymph nodes, and the pathologist will check each node for presence of cancer cells. Finding cancer cells in your axillary lymph nodes is a good predictor that the cancer has begun to spread beyond the breast.

One complication of extensive surgery in the armpit is damage to one or more of the nerves, either accidentally or because the injury was unavoidable. This may result in short or long term numbness in the armpit area, or weakness in some of the shoulder muscles. Often the numbness will improve over several years, but the sensitivity may not be normal. The weakness can generally be overcome with time.

Lymphedema

A more serious problem is a condition called *lymphedema*. Scarring of lymph vessels in the underarm area after removal of the lymph nodes may slow the circulation of lymph fluid, causing swelling of the arm, limiting its function, and making the arm more prone to infection. In advanced, untreated cases lymphedema can be a serious, debilitating problem.

As many as 10-20% of women undergoing axillary lymph node dissection will develop lymphedema of the arm. The condition may occur soon after surgery, or years later. In most cases it will be mild – you will notice some swelling in your fingers that may affect how you wear your rings. In women who are older, who are overweight, or who had radiation therapy, lymphedema is more likely to be more severe.

NINA-Nurse Navigator

The first sign that you are developing lymphedema might be a feeling of tightness in your watch band, or in your clothes. Or the fingers feel "full" when you try to make a fist. See your doctor immediately. Baseline measurements and early treatment with proper follow up might keep a serious problem from becoming a devastating condition.

How to reduce the risk of developing lymphedema

- Avoid cuts, burns, and insect bites.

- If your arm becomes red, swollen, or feels hot, call your doctor at once.

- Treat skin injuries promptly with anti-infection measures.

- Maintain a healthy body weight. Being overweight strains the lymphatic system.

- See a therapist to regain full strength and range of motion in the arm. This will improve lymph flow.

- Rest, inactivity, and being over-protective of the arm will not reduce the risk of lymphedema.

- It is acceptable to use the arm for blood drawing or to start IVs.

- It is acceptable to have the blood pressure checked on the limb where lymph nodes were removed. This does not raise the risk of developing lymphedema in that limb.

For women who develop lymphedema, the treatment will focus on lymph-draining massage, special compression bandages, and special exercises, all under the supervision of a qualified therapist.

Do you recommend that I
have a sentinel lymph
node biopsy instead of
a full axillary lymph
node dissection?

What are the reasons for
your recommendation?

Are you and your surgical
team experienced in
performing this proce-
dure?

SENTINEL LYMPH NODE BIOPSY

In an attempt to avoid the serious side effects of a full axillary lymph node dissection, a more refined technique was developed: *sentinel lymph node biopsy*. In many communities sentinel lymph node biopsy is considered the "standard of care".

The principle is simple. As lymphatic fluid drains away from the breast, it first passes through certain lymph nodes located in key parts of the drainage system. These are called **sentinel nodes**, because they act as guardians, or gatekeepers to the rest of the system. If the sentinel node is free of cancer cells, the odds are that there will be no cancer in the nodes located downstream. If cancer is found, a full dissection is done.

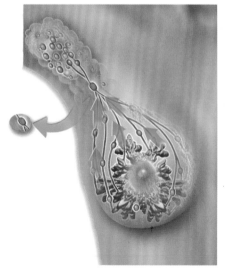

The sentinel lymph node biopsy begins with the injection of a blue dye and/or of a small amount of special material into the area near the tumor. The lymphatic fluid carries the materials to the first node in its path—the sentinel node. During surgery, the surgeon identifies and removes the sentinel node. If no cancer cells are found, a full dissection can be avoided.

A sentinel lymph node biopsy requires a surgeon who is experienced in the technique, but it helps avoid the potentially serious complications that can result from a full axillary lymph node dissection, particularly lymphedema.

*Lymphatic fluid drains through the sentinel
node, which is identified and removed
during surgery*

CHAPTER 5

RECONSTRUCTION

Why Breast Reconstruction?

Almost any woman who has had a mastectomy can have her breast reconstructed. New techniques and better skills enable surgeons to achieve results that can be remarkably natural and pleasing.

For many women, a breast reconstruction is an opportunity to regain their feminine silhouette, restore their self-image, and get on with their lives.

Today about three out of four women choose to have breast reconstruction after mastectomy. About half of them decide on implants. Most of the others prefer reconstruction with their own tissues.

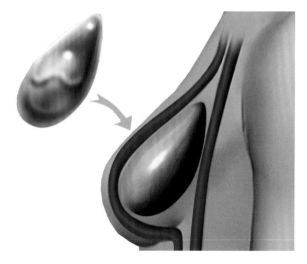

Breast reconstruction with implants is one of the many possible methods

Sadly, in some parts of the country, women are not offered the opportunity for immediate reconstruction. Even if your physician doesn't bring it up, or if you can't stand the thought of additional surgery, don't dismiss the possibility of rebuilding your breast, at the time of the mastectomy, or at a later date. Give it careful consideration. In the future, you might be glad you did.

Choosing a Plastic Surgeon

If you are considering reconstruction, even if it's to be done at a later date, arrange a meeting with a plastic surgeon well before your mastectomy, to discuss the details of the procedure.

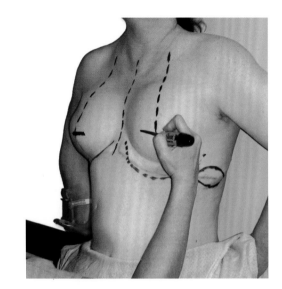

Breast reconstruction is not just science. It is also an art.

It is crucial that you select a surgeon who has extensive experience in reconstructive breast surgery, and is a board-certified specialist, because the cosmetic results will depend significantly on the surgeon's skill. Your primary surgeon can refer you to one.

Be sure to ask the surgeon who will perform your reconstruction to show you photos, and perhaps arrange for you to interview some of the patients who had the same procedure that you are considering. General surgeons who are trained in oncoplastic surgery techniques should be able to achieve good results with implant procedures, but be sure to check out their results first.

One more point: it is important that your expectations be realistic. The new breast may look natural, and may feel normal to someone touching it, but you will not have sensation in the nipple, and decreased or no sensation in the skin of the breast. Your satisfaction with the final result will depend as much on the surgeon's skill, as on your expectations.

Reconstruction Options

Reconstruction can be done at any time: at the time of mastectomy (*immediate reconstruction*) or at a later date (*delayed reconstruction*). Most women choose the immediate reconstruction option, which often yields better results.

There are several methods for reconstruction. One uses *synthetic implants* to create the shape of a breast. The other relies on the patient's own tissues, called *flaps*, transplanted from another area of the body.

Very commonly, you may need a minor plastic procedure on the other breast, such as a breast lift, to achieve the most symmetric look.

Reconstruction may be easier if you have a skin-sparing mastectomy, where much of the skin of the breast is left in place.

Once the breast is rebuilt, you can go on to have a reconstruction of the nipple and the areola, to achieve an even more natural look.

RECONSTRUCTION WITH IMPLANTS

The most common method of breast reconstruction is with implants. Implants are teardrop-shaped pouches that are inserted under the skin to create the form of a breast. The implant shell is made of silicone, and it is filled with saline (salt water solution) or with silicone gel. After extensive studies, most surgeons and oncologists are satisfied that today's silicone implants are safe.

Before your mastectomy, you will meet with a plastic surgeon to choose an implant that will match your other breast and provide a pleasing, symmetrical appearance. You may want to clip pictures of women's breasts to bring to the meeting as examples of what you would like.

If you're having immediate reconstruction, the plastic surgeon will take over right after the mastectomy, while you're still under anesthesia. This part of the surgery will take about an hour.

In order to achieve the most pleasant shape and feel for the reconstructed breast, the implant is usually placed *under* the muscle, rather than directly under the skin. Sometimes a patch made of biological material is used to reinforce the muscle and provide better coverage of the implant.

In another technique the implant is inserted *over* the muscle, directly *under* the skin, which results in less post-operative pain.

If the implant is small, and sufficient skin from the breast remains in place, the surgeon may be able to insert the implant without undue stretch to the skin and muscles of your chest wall. With this *single-stage procedure*, your reconstruction will be complete.

However, if the implant is too large, the surgeon will need to use a temporary expander to stretch and reshape the skin enough to accomodate the implant. This is called a *two-stage procedure*.

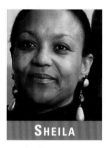

SHEILA

In the beginning, I started out with external prostheses. I didn't realize that I would end up with double D's again. These things are heavy! Wearing them eight hours gave me chest pain, backache, and headache, and so pretty soon, I began leaving them in the drawer, except when I needed to look "normal." And then I decided... "reconstruction."

JANET

It didn't seem that important at first, but finally having a reconstruction did wonders for my confidence. Now when I look in the mirror, I don't cringe. When I change in the locker room, I don't hide. In my own mind, I'm a woman again.

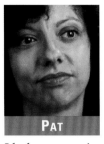

PAT

I had reconstruction at the time of the mastectomy. They put in an expander and slowly filled that for three months and then put in a permanent implant. I am very happy with it.

The expander is an elastic bag equipped with a fill tube and a valve. After the expander is inserted, it is filled with a small amount of saline. You'll return to the surgeon's office every week or two to have more saline injected into the expander. Gradually, over three to six months, the skin and muscle will stretch, just like they do over the abdomen during pregnancy.

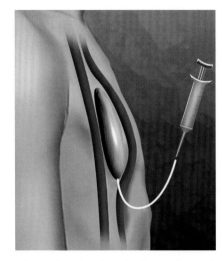

Expander placed under layer of muscle to achieve better results

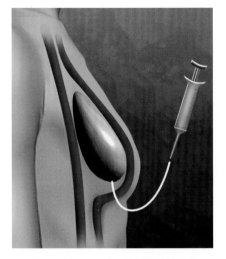

Expander gradually filled with saline over several weeks

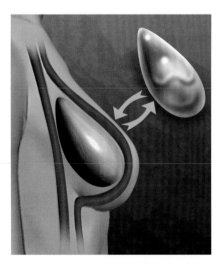

Expander replaced with implant in second-stage procedure

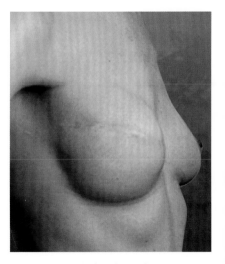

Completed implant reconstruction

In the second stage of the procedure, the expander is removed and the permanent implant is inserted. A nipple and areola can be created at a later date.

If you had a skin sparing mastectomy, your natural skin will provide the perfect pocket into which an implant can be placed.

You may also need additional surgery, such as a reduction, or a breast lift, on the other breast, to achieve the best symmetry possible.

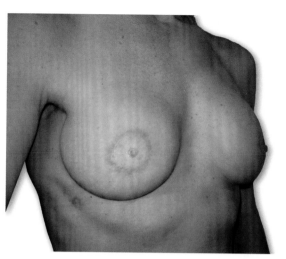

Symmetrical, natural looking reconstruction with implants. Next stage: tattooing of skin to enhance the areola

After Surgery

The first 24 to 72 hours after your initial implant surgery is when you experience the most discomfort. Your breast will be swollen and tender. Although every woman's recovery time is different, you should be able to resume many of your regular activities after about one week. You will need to wait at least one month before doing anything strenuous.

During the several weeks required to fully inflate the expander, you will probably have a feeling of fullness in your breast, but no major discomfort.

Over months, scar tissue forms around the implant, creating a tissue capsule. Most of the time, tissue capsules are soft and feel natural. However, in 15% of the cases, the capsule turns into a hard scar that distorts the breast, giving it the consistency of an orange. The surgeon can break up the scar tissue or replace the implant.

If your breast is treated with radiation therapy, the risk of scar tissue and hardening increases.

Most implants that have been in place for 10–15 years have some leakage. The body will react to the leak by forming a protective cyst around the leak. An MRI scan can spot even small amounts of leakage. If the leak leads to significant breast shrinkage, or change in shape, the implant will need to be replaced.

QUESTIONS TO ASK YOUR PLASTIC SURGEON:

What type of reconstruction do you think is best for me?

Will an implant make it more difficult to detect a local recurrence?

What should I know about the "skin-sparing" mastectomy?

Can you show me pictures of reconstruction procedures you have done?

Could I meet with some of the women so I can see and feel their breasts?

Will I have a lot of pain? How can the pain be treated?

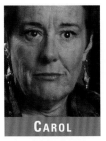

CAROL

One of the really good things about having reconstruction immediately, was that I woke up with a breast. Or something that passed for a breast, anyway. Now that it's healed, I can wear clothes that are tight or very low cut, and I don't have to worry about how I look.

SUSAN

I had the buttock flap, and wound up with a tiny scar on my behind that you can hardly see, and a firm breast. And as soon as I was out of the hospital, I went straight to lunch with a friend.

RECONSTRUCTION WITH YOUR OWN TISSUES

Breast reconstruction can be done using skin, muscle, and fat taken from another part of your body. This is also called an autologous reconstruction, myocutaneous flap, or simply, a *flap*.

There are different types of flaps. Some, (like TRAM flaps and latissimus dorsi flaps), move tissues from an area of the body to the breast area, while preserving the original blood supply. Others, (like the DIEP, SIEP, or IGAP) are *free flaps*—the blood supply to the transplanted tissue is cut, then reconstructed.

New types of flaps and flap procedures are being constantly developed and perfected. Ask your surgeon what is best for you.

TRAM and DIEP Flaps

The TRAM flap (Transverse Rectus Abdominis) uses one of the rectus abdominis muscles—the "abs," as weight lifters call them. The muscle, fat, and skin are separated from their natural attachments, and pulled up, under the skin, to the breast area. The flap is then shaped into the form of a breast. Some of the original blood supply is preserved. Rarely, a hernia may develop in the area from where the muscle was taken.

The DIEP flap (based on the Deep Inferior Epigastric Perforator artery) uses tissue from the same area as the TRAM flap, but only skin and fat, not the muscle or its blood supply.

TRAM and DIEP flaps are the most versatile of the tissue flaps, and can create a good match to the other breast for all but the largest-breasted women. An additional cosmetic benefit is that they also give the woman a "tummy tuck" as part of the procedure.

The procedures take three to five hours, and usually require a four to seven day hospital stay. They also entail an abdominal incision, and do result in significant discomfort for some time after the surgery. The procedures are complex, and should be performed only by plastic surgeons with extensive experience in this method.

Transverse Rectus Abdominis Flap

QUESTIONS TO ASK YOUR
INSURANCE COMPANY:

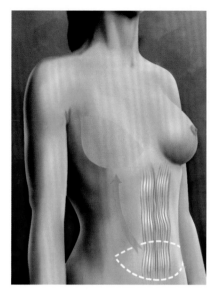

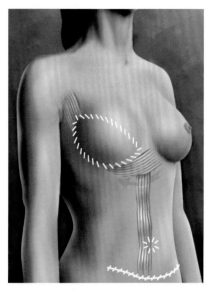

Tissue from the abdomen is used to create a breast mound

Does my policy cover the costs of the implant surgery, the implant anesthesia, and other related hospital costs? To what extent?

Does it cover plastic surgery on the other breast so I can look symmetric?

Does it cover removal of the implants if this becomes necessary?

If I choose to delay reconstruction and my company changes insurance plans, will I still be covered for breast reconstruction at a later date?

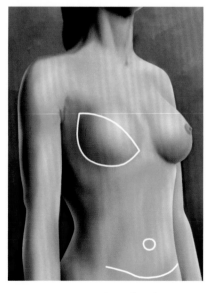

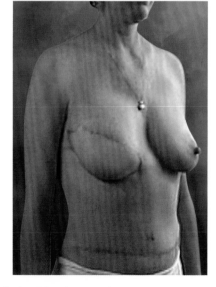

Completed reconstruction includes a "tummy tuck"

Latissimus Dorsi Flap

The latissimus dorsi flap is sometimes referred to as Lat flap. An incision is made under the shoulder blade, and a temporary tunnel is created under the skin, just like for the TRAM flap. A portion of the latissimus dorsi muscle from the upper back, and the fat and skin covering it, are pulled through this tunnel and relocated to the breast area. For most women, the latissimus muscle does not provide enough bulk to match the opposite breast, so a synthetic implant is added to make the reconstructed breast larger.

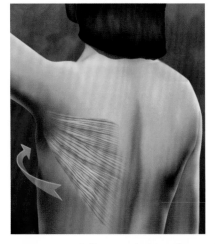 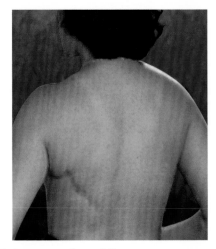

A flap consisting of part of the latissimus muscle and fat . . .

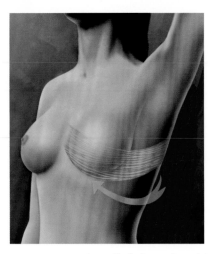 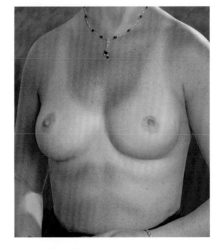

. . . is pulled through a skin tunnel to complete the reconstruction

Free Flaps

To create a free flap, tissue is removed from the abdomen or buttocks, and transplanted to the breast site. The original blood supply to the flap is cut, and then reconnected to a new artery and vein in the breast area. These procedures require a plastic surgeon who is skilled in micro-surgery, because they involve reconnecting blood vessels so thin, that the work must be done under a microscope.

Several free flaps use the so-called perforator vessels—blood vessels that branch off a deep artery and pass through the muscle, on the way to the fat and skin. The plastic surgeon isolates these vessels from the bigger artery, and dissects them out through the muscle, rather than taking them with the muscle.

This technique offers the benefit of a longer blood vessel that is easier to reattach in the breast area. By preserving the muscle at the donor site, the patient's recovery is shortened, and there is much less discomfort after surgery.

Free flaps include the DIEP flap and the IGAP flap. The IGAP or GAP flap uses the inferior gluteal artery and a portion of the buttock tissue. This way the location of the donor site can be effectively concealed, and the outline of the buttock preserved.

After Surgery

Your post-operative course will depend on the procedure you had, and on your body's ability to heal. For some of the more complex free flap procedures, you will spend 24 hours in the intensive care unit, where you will have frequent checks to ensure that the blood supply to the flap is adequate. Then you will be transferred to a regular floor to continue your convalescence.

The care of the wound will be almost the same as if you only had a mastectomy. You will have additional drains in place that will need to be drained by you or your caregiver several times a day.

YOLANDA

I went for the one with the perforating vessels. I had to stay in the hospital for four or five days. They watched the flap to make sure it was taking. But I was surprised that I was able to drive pretty much as soon as I got home. And the breast looks great!

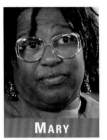

MARY

I have a lot of strong feelings about man-made
products in my body and
if I can't use the tissues
from my own body, I
don't think I will ever
have reconstruction.

All flap reconstructions are complicated procedures and involve certain risks. Large portions of tissues are moved, and their blood supply is disrupted. Sometimes the blood vessels get clogged and the flap may necrose, or die. This would require removal of the flap, causing significant discomfort and possible deformity.

Flaps cause pain both at the donor site and in the breast area. Removal of muscles from their original position can cause pain and weakness, or rarely, a hernia in the donor area. Naturally, you will have additional scars besides the ones on your breast.

On the other hand, the use of flaps avoids placing foreign materials into your body, and can result in the most natural-looking reconstructions. Many women—and their partners—appreciate the fact that the breast feels more natural than after an implant reconstruction.

Nipple and Areola Reconstruction

Women who want their reconstructed breast to look as natural as possible may choose to have a nipple and areola reconstruction. This procedure is usually done a few months after the breast reconstruction, so that the breast has had time to settle into its natural sag.

Small flaps of skin on the reconstructed breast are raised and brought togeth-er into the shape of a nipple. The areola is created either from a skin graft, or by tattooing. The procedures can be done under local anesthesia.

Note that the new nipples will always be erect, and will not be sensitive. If you prefer, you can buy plastic removable nipples that come in semi-erect form. They are surprisingly lifelike in texture and color.

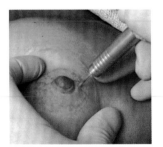

*The areola is created
by tattooing the skin*

WHICH IS RIGHT FOR ME?

You have many options for breast reconstruction. Here are some factors to keep in mind when making your decisions:

Synthetic Implants:

• Implants can be easily placed by most plastic surgeons.
• There is less surgery, less pain, shorter recovery, no additional scar, and less expense than with tissue flaps.
• They are not lifetime devices, and may rupture or need replacement.
• Implants may lead to hardening and misplacement.

Tissue Flaps:

• They are typically soft and normal-appearing.
• There is no artificial implant in the body.
• With some flaps, a "tummy tuck" is an added bonus.
• There is lengthy, extensive, and expensive surgery, with blood transfusions and considerable post-operative discomfort.
• There is an additional scar at the donor site.
• There is a risk of the flap "not taking."

Immediate Reconstruction:

• You don't have to wake up from mastectomy surgery without a breast.
• One surgery rather than two means lower cost, fewer problems from anesthetic and surgery, and less recovery time.

Delayed Reconstruction:

• Provides additional time to make reconstructive choices.
• For the woman undergoing chemotherapy, possibly decreases the chance of infection in the reconstruction area.

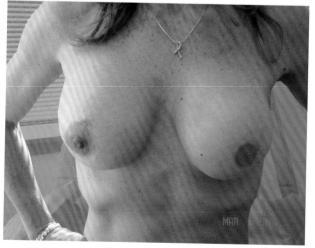

Beautiful reconstruction (her left breast) can be achieved by a surgeon trained in oncoplastic techniques

> **NINA-Nurse Navigator**
>
> You can expect better results if the reconstruction is done immediately, at the time of the surgery. But all is not lost if you decide down the line that you want it. It is still possible.

EVELYN

I think when I had my
surgery, I wasn't sure that I
wanted reconstruction. It
happened so fast. I probably should have asked for a
consultation with a plastic
surgeon.

EXTERNAL BREAST FORMS

Many women choose to have no reconstruction of any type after the mas-
tectomy. Some make this decision because they want to avoid extra surgery.
Others because they're comfortable with their appearance and body image.
A few view their scars as battle scars from a war they waged.

If you choose to have no reconstruction, you may want to use a breast form
instead. Breast forms, or *prostheses* as they are also called, are available in a
variety of sizes, shapes, and colors. Some are designed to fit into a special
bra. Others can be attached securely to your chest using a special adhesive.
Prostheses range from inexpensive foam inserts to custom-molded replace-
ments with realistic color and texture, designed to duplicate your natural
breast as closely as possible.

Breast forms are used not just for appearance. They play an important function by relieving the uneven strain on your posture that may occur after a
mastectomy, particularly if your breasts are large.

The decision about whether to have breast reconstruction, or to wear an
external prosthesis instead, is a very personal one. It should be based on your
own feelings about your body, your sexuality, and your tolerance for additional surgery. Your decision is legitimate, and must be respected by your
healthcare providers and your loved ones.

CHAPTER 6

RADIATION THERAPY

What is Radiation Therapy?

Radiation therapy uses high-energy beams to destroy cancer cells. The beams resemble the X-rays that are used to create an image of the chest, or of a broken bone, but for treatment purposes, the rays are of much higher intensity.

The purpose of giving radiation therapy after a tumor was surgically removed, is to destroy any cancer cells that might remain in the breast area in order to prevent a recurrence.

Radiation beams are directed from several angles.

There are several ways to administer radiation therapy. ***External beam radiation therapy***, or EBRT, is the oldest. It uses a device called a linear accelerator to aim the treatment beam at the whole breast area from several angles. It is also known as *WBI*, or ***whole breast irradiation***.

Internal radiation, or ***brachytherapy***, relies on a radioactive source placed temporarily directly into the breast, to treat mostly the tissues around the tumor cavity.

Intraoperative radiation therapy, or IORT, uses a single large dose of radiation delivered in the operating room, at the time of surgery.

IORT and brachytherapy are referred to as *PBI*, or ***partial breast irradiation***.

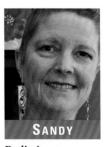

SANDY

Radiation was very easy for me – I thought I would have a skin burn, since I am fair skinned, but I didn't burn at all. When I came in for treatments, I was in there for just a few minutes, so it was no big deal, and it just became part of my daily routine.

Who Should Receive Radiation Therapy?

Years ago studies showed that a lumpectomy was as effective as a mastectomy, but only if the lumpectomy was combined with radiation therapy.

Today, lumpectomy is almost always followed by radiation therapy, with some exceptions. If you have already received radiation to that area of the body; if you have scleroderma, vasculitis or extra sensitive skin; or if you are pregnant, then radiation therapy may not be used.

In addition, for women who are over 70, and whose cancers are early-stage, not aggressive, and had good margins after lumpectomy, the benefit might be minimal as long as they remain on endocrine therapy.

EXTERNAL BEAM RADIATION THERAPY

Treatment Planning

The goal of radiation therapy is to deliver the optimal dose of cancer-damaging radiation to the breast area, with the least impact on the surrounding normal tissues. This requires a plan carefully tailored to each case.

Using a CT scanner, the radiation oncology team will determine the best angles for the beam. They will outline the treatment ports—places on your body where the beam will be aimed—and mark them with colored ink or tiny tattoos. These markings will ensure that the beam is aimed accurately every treatment session. Sometimes a special cast will be fabricated for your chest to ensure consistent positioning. Once the planning is completed, the treatments can begin.

How Treatment is Given

The treatment is given in a room with thick concrete walls and lead-lined doors, to protect those who are outside the treatment area from radiation. The device used to deliver radiation may seem complex and intimidating. But don't be alarmed. A TV monitor lets the staff keep you in sight at all times, in case you need anything.

The radiation therapist will adjust the position of the machine according to the previously determined settings, then step out of the room. The unit will be repositioned one or two times to change the angle of the beam. Each exposure lasts only a few minutes and you won't see or feel anything.

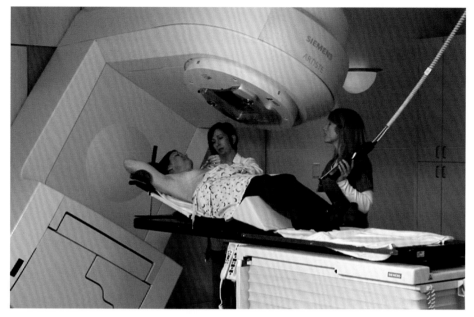

External Beam Radiation Therapy is delivered by a linear accelerator

How Long is the Full Course of External Beam Radiation Treatment?

Until recently, the standard full course of treatment was about five to seven weeks, with sessions from Monday through Friday. This schedule is a burden to women who have full time jobs or live far from the hospital.

Based on recent research, the new guidelines state that a method called *hypofractionation* is as effective for most cancers. A full therapeutic dose is delivered in three-to-five weeks, rather than five-to-seven, using slightly higher fractions. This offers patients a more convenient and lower cost option for their treatment, without compromising the likelihood that their cancer will return or increasing their risk of side effects.

The start of your therapy will depend on whether you are also undergoing chemotherapy. You may have chemotherapy and radiation therapy simultaneously, or be started on chemotherapy, then treated with radiation, then again with chemotherapy.

During the final week you may also receive an additional dose of radiation, called the "boost". The boost may be done with a different form of radiation, called an *electron beam*.

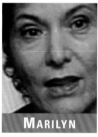

MARILYN

Cosmetically, I had very good results from the treatment. If you look at my breasts right now, you couldn't tell that there was treatment done to one breast as opposed to the other breast. They look exactly the same.

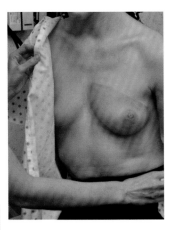

*Skin redness caused
by radiation*

**QUESTIONS TO ASK
YOUR DOCTOR:**

Why do I need radiation therapy?

Which method is better for me, external beam or brachytherapy?

Can I continue my usual work or exercise schedule?

Can I miss a few treatments?

Can I arrange to be treated elsewhere if I'm traveling?

What side effects, if they occur, should I report immediately?

Will I be able to conceive and bear a child after treatments?

What about the different cost of brachytherapy vs. external beam?

Side Effects of External Beam Radiation Therapy

Radiation therapy is a safe, proven treatment with few unwanted side effects. The most common are fatigue and skin changes. You will not have nausea or lose your hair, as you might with chemotherapy, and you certainly won't be radioactive. Most people find that they can go through radiation therapy while maintaining their normal lifestyle.

Fatigue. Most people begin to feel tired after a few weeks of radiation therapy, as a result of daily trips for treatment and the effects of radiation on normal cells. If you feel tired, limit your activities, use your leisure time in a restful way, and try to get more sleep at night. If you continue working, talk with your employer about adjusting your work schedule, or working from home.

Skin Changes. The energy waves used in radiation therapy have an effect on the skin that resembles the effect of intense sunlight. Some skin irritation and redness, similar to a sunburn, may develop by the third or fourth week of treatment. Don't rub or scratch the affected area. Use mild soap, being careful not to wash off port markings, if you have any. Wear soft clothing, preferably cotton, and protect the treated area from sunlight.

Breast Changes. Radiation therapy may cause breast swelling and tenderness, so you may find sleeping on your stomach uncomfortable. Try using pillows to create a comfortable position. The swelling will subside after treatment. On a long term basis, the breast may become slightly smaller or larger. The breast may also become slightly firmer, but significant hardening is rare.

What to Avoid During Radiation Therapy

Certain vitamins, such as vitamins C, A, D, and E, have antioxidant properties that help cells heal. However, this healing works against the action of radiation therapy, which works by damaging cancer cells.

A well-balanced diet will give you all the vitamins that you need in amounts that will not interfere with the treatment. You can resume the supplements after you complete your course of radiation therapy.

BRACHYTHERAPY

Another method of delivering radiation therapy is *brachytherapy.* Instead of an external beam, brachytherapy uses a temporary catheter and a radioactive source placed briefly into the tumor cavity. A computerized program ensures that the entire area receives an even dose of radiation, with minimal damage to normal tissues.

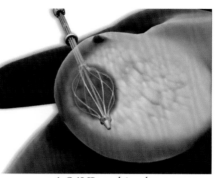

A SAVI multicatheter device within the breast

The treatment is repeated twice a day for five days. You are free to leave the hospital between treatments. This faster radiation technique, applied to a selected part of the breast is also called *accelerated partial breast irradiation,* or *APBI.* The time commitment required is shorter, and some patients find it more convenient.

INTRAOPERATIVE RADIATION THERAPY

In a technique called *intraoperative radiation therapy,* or *IORT,* the radiation is aimed directly at the area from where the tumor was removed, while surrounding healthy tissue is moved aside.

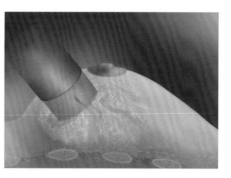

Mobetron device treating tumor cavity

The advantage of this method is that it delivers the entire radiation treatment in a single dose, while you are still in surgery. Depending on the facility, you may still need external beam radiation for a few weeks. But potentially, the long weeks of external beam radiation therapy may be reduced to about four to five minutes.

Internal vs. External vs. Intraoperative Radiation Therapy

Studies have shown that for select cases of breast cancer, **brachytherapy, intraoperative therapy, and external beam therapy are similarly effective** in destroying cancer cells within the breast, and reducing the chance of local cancer recurrence.

For some women, shorter schedules may have significant advantages. Women who would have to travel to a radiation therapy facility daily for five to seven weeks, can instead complete a course of treatment in days (hypofractionation) or even minutes (intraoperative).

The importance of this abbreviated treatment is enormous: reducing commuting time may make the difference between choosing lumpectomy with radiation, or settling for a mastectomy.

CHAPTER 7

CHEMOTHERAPY

Why Additional Therapy?

MRI, CT, PET scans, blood tests… All your tests came back "negative". So why would you need any therapy in addition to the surgery, if there are no signs of tumor spread to distant organs in your body?

The problem with cancer is that it can *metastasize*: as the tumor grows, cancer cells can break away and travel down blood vessels or lymph ducts to other parts of the body—much the same way as seeds from a weed are carried away by the wind, or float down a river, to sprout somewhere else.

In the very early stages, these groups of break-away cells, called *micrometastases*, are very small, and cannot be found by any test or method that exists today. With time, these tiny cancerous clumps will grow into larger tumors (metastases). If one postpones therapy until the metastases are large enough to be confirmed by imaging studies, the possibility of successful treatment decreases.

So if there is any reason to suspect that cells from your tumor had a chance to metastasize to other parts of your body before the cancer was removed, you may be treated with a systemic treatment such as chemotherapy, hormonal therapy or a targeted therapy, to destroy those tumor cells as soon as possible.

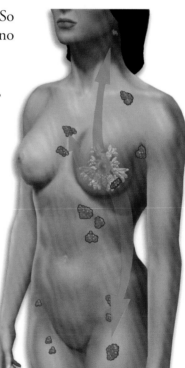

Early cancer metastases might be invisible to scans and tests

WHAT IS CHEMOTHERAPY?

Chemotherapy uses drugs, called cytotoxic (cell-killing) drugs, to destroy cancer cells. These drugs travel through the bloodstream to reach cancer cells almost anywhere in the body. Chemotherapy can be useful in a variety of situations.

Adjuvant chemotherapy is used after surgery as an additional tool to target any cancer cells that might have spread beyond the breast area.

Neo-adjuvant chemotherapy can be given before surgery to shrink a tumor so it can be removed with breast conserving surgery instead of a mastectomy. Pre-surgical use of chemotherapy can also test whether the tumor responds to a particular drug. If the tumor does not shrink, another chemotherapy can be tried, or your physician may proceed to surgery.

For *advanced* breast cancer in women whose cancer has spread outside the breast and underarm area.

HOW CHEMOTHERAPY WORKS

Cells go through several steps in the process of cell division. Chemotherapy drugs interfere with various parts of this cycle, making it difficult for the cells to reproduce and for the tumor to grow.

Chemotherapy affects rapidly dividing cells more effectively than slower dividing cells. Both normal cells (hair follicles, bone marrow, GI tract) and cancer cells are damaged, but because cancer cells generally divide more rapidly, and are less effective at self-repair, they are more likely to be destroyed than normal cells.

There are dozens of different chemotherapy drugs, each designed to interfere with a different part of the cell's duplication process. By using a combination of two or three different drugs, it is possible to affect several phases of the duplication cycle and increase the effectiveness of the treatment.

Recent advances in *genomic testing* (analysis of the genetic make up of your cancer cells) are enabling scientists to predict with more accuracy how your tumor might respond to various drugs.

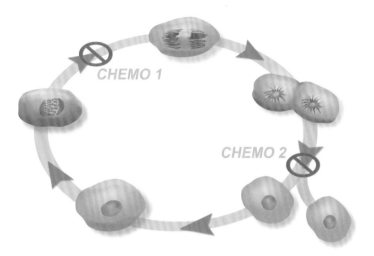

Different chemotherapy drugs disrupt different parts of the cell division cycle

Your oncologist will recommend the best drug or combination of drugs, based on the characteristics of your tumor, degree of suspected spread, and your general health.

Since some drug combinations are more likely than others to put you into early menopause, or make it difficult for you to have children in the future, you may want to discuss the drug selection in detail.

HOW CHEMOTHERAPY IS GIVEN

Most chemotherapy drugs are given by injection into a vein (intravenously, or IV). The injections can be done in a private doctor's office, in a hospital, or in a cancer center. A few chemotherapy drugs are given orally, and you take them at home.

Chemotherapy is given in cycles. Each cycle may be as short as one week, or as long as four weeks. This allows the normal cells in your body to recover between treatments. The full course of therapy can be four to six or more cycles, over three to six months. Chemotherapy typically begins as soon as possible after surgery.

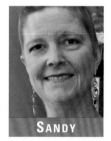

SANDY

When chemo was mentioned, I told myself that I wasn't going to be sick, and that was that. And I wasn't. I never threw up – not once.

QUESTIONS TO ASK
YOUR DOCTOR:

Do I need chemo-
therapy? Why?

What drugs do you
recommend?

What are the benefits and
risks of chemotherapy?

How successful is this
treatment for the type
of cancer I have?

How will you evaluate the
effectiveness of the
treatments?

What side effects will I
experience?

Can I work while I'm hav-
ing chemotherapy?

Can I travel between treatments (short business
or pleasure trips)?

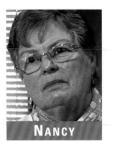

NANCY

My oncologist discussed the
choice of chemo with the
whole team at the breast center. It was very comforting
that it wasn't just one person
deciding. It was the group.

In a method called ***dose-dense chemotherapy***, drugs are given more frequently – for example, every two weeks, instead of every three. Studies have
shown that by reducing the interval between doses, it is possible to improve
the outcome of the treatment in women whose cancers have spread to lymph
nodes.

The decreased interval between doses gives your normal cells less time to
recover between treatments. As a result, your blood cell count may drop.
Your medical team may prescribe medications that help stimulate the bone
marrow to produce more blood cells.

Do not confuse "dose-dense chemotherapy" with "bone marrow trans-
plants". In this procedure, now obsolete, bone marrow cells were harvested,
preserved by freezing, then re-implanted after high doses of chemotherapy.
The procedure was complex and expensive, and recent studies have shown
that it has no advantages over conventional treatment.

An IV Chemo Day

Healthcare professionals realize that chemotherapy may be a stressful experience for you, and try to make your visit as pleasant as possible. Many facilities strive to create cozy, relaxed and friendly environments.

You may make friends with some of the other patients who come for treatment at the same time. Bring an iPad or a book, or practice relaxation to
make the session more pleasant. Depending on how you feel after treatments, you may want to ask a friend to come with you—for company, or to
drive you home.

Before you receive the scheduled dose of chemotherapy, the nurse will draw
your blood, to check whether the blood-producing cells in your bone marrow have adequately recovered, and to verify whether chemotherapy is
affecting your liver or other organs. If the results of the tests are outside of
normal limits, your oncologist may decide to lower the dose of chemo, or
postpone the treatment.

If your results are acceptable, the nurse will take you to the treatment area
and start the IV (intravenous line) through which the drug will be injected.

If your veins are easy to reach, this will take a few seconds, and feel like a pinprick. Then the drug will be administered. Some drugs are given as a rapid injection, others are dripped in slowly over a longer period—sometimes up to three hours. Generally you won't feel any discomfort.

Vascular Access Devices

Sometimes veins are thin, damaged, or covered by a layer of fat, making it difficult for the nurse to start an IV line. In addition, a few chemo drugs can be very irritating to the veins, and can damage the vein at the injection site. In such cases a port may be installed under the skin.

A port consists of a tube (catheter), attached to a dome-shaped chamber. The device is surgically implanted under the skin, with the dome placed in the chest or arm. The catheter is threaded into a large vein, where rapid blood flow will dilute the drug, and keep it from damaging the lining of the vein. The whole device will be completely covered by skin, so it will not interfere with your activities. You can swim, bathe and exercise freely.

Ports can also be used by port-trained staff for drawing blood, thus avoiding needle sticks of the arms during clinic visits.

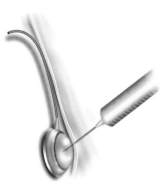

Chemotherapy drugs injected through a port

SIDE EFFECTS OF CHEMOTHERAPY

When first told that they have breast cancer, many women panic at the thought of having to go through chemotherapy, because they have heard of chemotherapy as something that makes you deathly ill, or makes your hair fall out. "Will I have to have chemo?" is one of the first questions that many women ask.

Much has changed in recent years. Today there are very effective drugs that can greatly reduce—and sometimes eliminate—the side effects of chemotherapy, making the experience much more tolerable than it was rumored to be in the past.

Why do chemotherapy drugs cause side effects? Besides damaging cancer cells, chemotherapy affects all rapidly dividing cells such as the gastrointestinal or GI tract, the bone marrow, hair follicles and the reproductive system.

MARILYN

I actually did some modeling during the time I was on chemotherapy, which is sort of a contradiction in terms for many people. But, it really got me through what might have been a difficult period and it made it a very positive year for me.

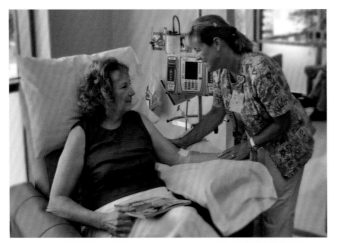

The staff will make you as comfortable as possible during chemotherapy treatment

So the most common side effects are related to these organs, and include nausea, fatigue, menopausal symptoms and hair loss. The side effects will vary with the drug used, and with your own tolerance to it.

Be prepared for possible side effects, but don't assume that you will have all, many, or even a few of them. Many people go through chemotherapy without significant ill effects.

Don't compare your treatment with that of another patient, because there are so many different varieties of breast cancer. Your treatment will have been personalized for your particular case. And remember, if you don't have side effects, it does not mean that the drugs are not working.

It's not likely that you will ever look forward to your chemotherapy days, but a positive attitude, help from your healthcare team, and support from your friends and family can make chemotherapy a tolerable experience.

Nausea

Today, thanks to powerful antiemetic drugs, nausea is much less common than in years past. There are several effective medications available that will control, if not completely eliminate, nausea. Discuss this with your healthcare professionals, and make sure that you are receiving the best anti-nausea medication for your particular needs. Remember, effective control of nausea may make the difference between completing the full course of therapy, or quitting too early and running the risk of developing metastatic cancer. In addition to medications, consider other options, such as relaxation or imagery, that have proven to be quite effective for many patients. You can find more information on this subject in Chapter 9.

Nausea can lead to loss of appetite. Since good nutrition is very important to help you fight cancer and retain strength, you should make sure that you have adequate food intake, especially proteins and fluids. Eat small frequent meals and avoid stomach-bloating carbonated liquids.

NINA-Nurse Navigator

Most patients tell me that chemo wasn't as bad as they initially thought it would be. For most, the nausea and tiredness wasn't bad at all. They worried about their hair falling out but once it did, it was almost a sense of relief knowing that they passed this point in their treatment.

A few simple steps that can relieve nausea:

- Eat foods that made you feel better in the past, like ginger ale or crackers.

- Remove dentures on days you receive drug treatments.

- Wear loose clothing.

- Try breathing through your mouth when you feel nauseated.

- Avoid fried or other fatty foods.

- Hold a mint or lemon drop in your mouth.

- Avoid eating your favorite foods when you are nauseated, so that you do not develop an aversion to them.

- If the smell of food makes you nauseated, cook outside or take a walk while the food is being prepared.

CHARLENE

My physician had given me several different anti-emetics to find the absolute best for me to combat the nausea and vomiting. I will say that it definitely was trial and error. Some did not work for me, others helped a lot.

If you do experience nausea, it usually won't be until hours or even days after the infusion. It may last from a few hours to up to several days, depending on the individual person. In rare instances, the nausea can be severe.

Despite the possible loss of appetite, many women notice an increase in weight as a result of treatment with most chemotherapy drugs. Weight gain of up to twenty pounds is not uncommon, and can be a distressing side effect. For the sake of maintaining your well being, be cautious of any weight gain.

Fatigue

Chemotherapy can make you feel tired, especially on the first day after each treatment. Adjust your schedule so that you can rest if you want.

Many women find that they can keep a fairly normal level of activity. If you feel totally unable to function at a reasonable level, tell your oncologist about it. Your drug dose may be too high, and may need to be adjusted. In addition, your physician may recommend medications to help your body rebuild red blood cells, which may increase your energy level.

NINA-Nurse Navigator

Interestingly, the best antidote to fatigue is exercise. Make a point of doing something physical every day, even if it is only a short walk around the yard. You'll feel stronger and more empowered.

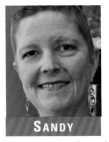

SANDY

My energy level was low for two or three days after the treatment, but never so that I couldn't get out of bed. A few days into the cycle I could do pretty much whatever I wanted.

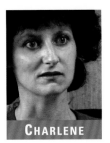

CHARLENE

The absolute very worst was the hair loss. That did me in. When I was in the shower, all of a sudden it would just come out in my hand, crops of it. Once it was gone, I felt relieved.

After your first or second cycles, you will have a good idea of what to expect. Ask your healthcare team to help you anticipate your "good days" and your "bad days", so you can optimize your time. For example, mark your "chemo days" on your calendar. Avoid important business appointments during the first week, when you are likely to feel the worst. Try scheduling the family get away for the third week, when you can expect to feel your best.

Hair Loss

One of the side effects of chemotherapy that causes women the most distress is hair loss. How much hair you lose—some or all—will depend on which drugs you are getting. The good news is that hair lost due to chemotherapy always grows back, sometimes thicker than it was originally.

Usually hair falls out over a period of a few weeks, starting around the third week after the first dose of chemotherapy. You may find large clumps on your pillow, or in the shower, or notice a lot of hair in your comb. Some women experience a sudden loss of hair.

Buy a wig before your hair falls out, and try to pick one that resembles your natural hair. Insurance may cover some of the cost. Ask your beautician to style your wig the way you usually wear your hair.

Look Good...Feel Better is a public service program sponsored by the Cosmetic, Toiletry, and Fragrance Association Foundation in partnership with the American Cancer Society and the National Cosmetology Association. The program helps women manage changes in their appearance resulting from cancer treatment.

Mouth sores and intestinal problems

The mouth, stomach, and intestines are lined with cells that divide relatively rapidly. Anti-cancer drugs can affect these organs, leading to mouth sores and diarrhea. Do not take any over-the-counter medications unless specifically recommended by your health care provider.

It is a good idea to see your dentist before you begin chemotherapy to take care of any pre-existing problems such as cavities or abscesses. Ask your dentist to advise you on how to brush and floss during chemotherapy.

Let your physician know if you experience tooth issues during the treatment. Some chemo drugs may lead to bone loss including in the jaw, which may cause your teeth to become lose.

Oral care during cancer treatment:

- Eat foods cold or at room temperature.

- Choose soft, soothing foods, such as ice cream, milkshakes, baby food, etc. You also can puree cooked foods.

- Avoid irritating, acidic foods, such as tomatoes, or citrus fruit, spicy or salty foods; and rough, coarse, or dry foods.

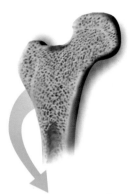

Bone marrow produces...

Maintaining good mouth care and using a soft toothbrush will help minimize sores. If sores do develop, you may find that frozen juices, ice cream, and watermelon can be very soothing. If your mouth gets dry, ask your doctor if you should use an artificial saliva product to moisten your mouth. Suck on ice chips, popsicles, or sugarless hard candy. Moisten dry foods with butter, margarine, gravy or sauce.

Bone Marrow Suppression

Bone marrow cells, which produce red blood cells, white blood cells, and platelets in your blood, are strongly affected by chemotherapy, and may lose some, or all, of their function. This will lead to lower blood cell counts. Red blood cells (RBC's) transport oxygen. The normal value, measured in mg (milligrams) of hemoglobin (Hb, the oxygen carrying protein in the cell) is twelve to fourteen. A low red blood cell count, called anemia, will generally give you fatigue.

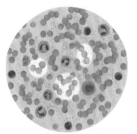

red blood cells,

White blood cells (WBC's) help fight infection. A normal WBC count is in the 4,000-10,000 range. There are several different types of white blood cells. The most important for fighting infection are called neutrophils. Oncologists use the absolute neutrophil count (ANC) to monitor patients under treatment, and to determine whether the next dose can be given. A neutrophil count of less than 1000 is called neutropenia, and makes you susceptible to colds or infections, including skin wound infections.

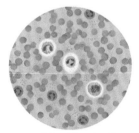

white blood cells,

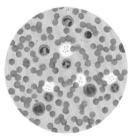

and platelets

NINA-Nurse Navigator

Take control of your upcoming hair loss. Try shorter styles that you have always wanted to try. Color your hair a color that would otherwise be too bold for you. Take charge and make it your own.

Platelets help the blood clot. A low platelet count, below 150,000, can predispose to bleeding. This can take the form of easy bruising, excessive bleeding from wounds, or slow bleeding into the stomach or intestine, which could appear as black stools.

Your chemotherapy dose will be adjusted to achieve the maximum effect on the tumor cells, without dangerously impairing the ability of the bone marrow to produce blood cells in sufficient quantities.

If your bone marrow becomes excessively suppressed, your doctor may add other

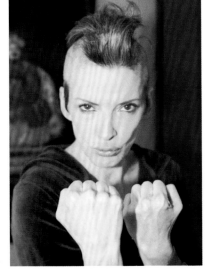

Lou Gideon

medications to your treatment, to stimulate your bone marrow to produce more blood cells. Raising your white cell count will help you fight off infections. Raising your red cell count will give your blood more capacity to carry oxygen, and will improve your strength.

Infections

When your white blood cell count is low, your body may not be able to fight off infections, even if you take extra care. Most infections come from bacteria normally found on the skin, in the intestines, and in the genital tract.

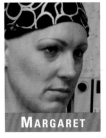

MARGARET

I had contacted my beautician and got two wigs before the hair came out. So the first day, as soon as it started falling, I had the wigs on. And the wigs have been just fine.

Signs that you might have an infection

- Fever over 100 degrees Fahrenheit
- Sweating and chills
- Loose bowels
- A burning feeling when you urinate
- A severe cough or sore throat
- Unusual vaginal discharge or itching
- Redness, swelling, or tenderness around a wound

Report any signs of infection to your doctor right away. This is especially important when your white blood cell count is low. If you have a fever, don't use aspirin, acetaminophen (Tylenol), or any other medicine to bring your temperature down without first checking with your doctor.

Prevent infections when your white count is down

- Wash your hands often. Be sure to wash them extra well before you eat and before and after you use the bathroom.

- Clean your rectal area thoroughly after each bowel movement. Check with your doctor before using enemas or suppositories.

- Stay away from people who have diseases you can catch, such as a cold, the flu, measles, or chickenpox. Try to avoid crowds.

- Stay away from children who recently have received immunizations, such as vaccines for polio, measles or mumps.

- Don't cut or tear the cuticles off your nails.

- Be careful not to nick yourself when using sharp tools.

- Use an electric shaver instead of a razor to prevent cuts.

- Use a soft toothbrush that won't hurt your gums.

- Take a warm (not hot) bath, shower, or sponge bath every day. Pat your skin dry using a light touch. Don't rub.

- Clean cuts and scrapes right away with water and an antiseptic.

- Wear protective gloves when gardening or cleaning up after animals and others, especially small children.

- Do not get any immunization shots without checking with your doctor first.

QUESTIONS TO ASK YOUR DOCTOR:

How can I manage nausea?

Will I be given medications to treat side effects?

Can I take public transportation home after treatments?

Should I eat before I come for my treatments?

Can I take vitamins or herbs if I choose?

QUESTIONS TO ASK
YOUR DOCTOR:

Will I continue to have my
menstrual periods?

If not, when will they
return?

Should I use birth
control? What type do
you recommend?

Will I be able to conceive
and bear a child after
treatments?

OTHER SIDE EFFECTS

"Chemo brain"

Another possible side effect of chemotherapy is "chemo brain." Many women experience a slight decrease in mental functioning, such as problems with concentration and memory. These may last a long time. Although many women have blamed this on chemotherapy, it also has been seen in women who were not treated with chemotherapy.

Sexual Side Effects—Physical

Chemotherapy often suppresses a woman's ovarian function, reducing the amount of estrogen in the body, and causing menopause-like symptoms such as hot flashes and vaginal dryness.

Ask your doctor or nurse to recommend a suitable non-estrogen treatment to help reduce hot flashes. Use a vaginal lubricant if necessary to manage any discomfort during intercourse. To help prevent infection, avoid oil-based lubricants such as petroleum jelly, wear cotton underwear and pantyhose with a ventilated cotton lining, and don't wear tight slacks or shorts.

Doctors advise women of childbearing age to use birth control throughout their treatment, because anti-cancer drugs may cause birth defects. If a woman is pregnant when her cancer is discovered, it may be possible to delay chemotherapy until after the baby is born, or until after the twelfth week of pregnancy, when the fetus is beyond the stage of greatest risk.

Chemotherapy may also make it more difficult to conceive. If a woman is young, and would like to have children after cancer treatment, it is now possible to harvest eggs from her ovaries, and preserve them by freezing. After treatment, the eggs can be fertilized in vitro and implanted into the woman's womb.

Egg harvesting is a difficult procedure, and may delay chemotherapy. In addition, the hormones used in harvesting and the hormonal changes due to the pregnancy may have undesirable effects on the breast cancer. Discuss these serious issues with your physician.

NINA-Nurse Navigator

As you go through your treatments, you may not feel like being as intimate as usual. You might feel like you just need to be needed, or you might want reassurance. Communicate with your partner and be honest. Whatever you're feeling, talking through your concerns will help keep you close.

Sexual Side Effects—Psychological

During cancer treatment, many women find that their sexual interest declines because of the physical and emotional stresses. Don't be shy about discussing sexual issues with your nurse or doctor. They can offer a wealth of advice on how to handle any difficulties you may be facing, and help improve your quality of life.

If you and your partner find it difficult to talk to each other about sex, or cancer, or both, you may want to seek out a counselor who can help you communicate more openly.

An occasional romantic getaway to do something both of you enjoy may be a good aphrodisiac.

In Chapter 13 of this book we will discuss in greater detail how you can deal with this issue.

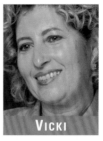

VICKI

Every chemo cycle made me feel worse and worse. So by the eighth round, I said, "Can I take a break please?" And that was fine with them, so I went on to have my radiation therapy and get that out of the way, then came back for the last two chemo cycles. So I finished the whole treatment.

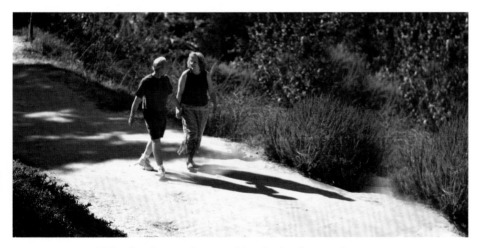

Take the time to do something both of you enjoy

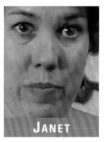

JANET

What seems to happen a lot of times with chemo, just like with menopause, is that your vagina shrinks and shortens. And you can have problems with dryness. That's the straw that breaks the camel's back sometimes. It's too embarrassing to even think about, let alone talk to anybody.

COMMON CHEMOTHERAPY DRUGS

There are dozens of drugs currently used for breast cancer treatment. Most are used in combinations of two, three, or more. Don't be confused because your doctor, nurse and pharmacist may refer to the drugs by different names. **Generic name** is the chemical name of the drug. **Brand name** is the name each manufacturer gives to their specific form of the same chemical. For example, the chemical compound called fluorouracil (its generic name) is marketed as 5-FU by one company, and as Adrucil by another.

The most common drugs used for breast cancer are cyclophosphamide, methotrexate, fluorouracil (5-FU), Adriamycin, and the taxane drugs Taxol and Taxotere. Drugs are often given in combination. For example, CMF—which stands for cyclophosphamide, methotrexate, and fluorouracil; CAF: cyclophosphamide, Adriamycin, and 5-fluorouracil; AC—for Adriamycin, and cyclophosphamide; or TAC—Taxotere, Adriamycin and Cytoxan.

You may want to write down the specific details about the drugs that you will be taking. Don't forget that your symptoms may not be the same as another patient's. And if you don't have symptoms, it doesn't mean the drugs are not working.

PAT

While I was on chemotherapy, I felt that I was actually doing something to take charge of the cancer, to kill any cancer cells that might be running amuck in my body. When I walked out of the chemo suite for the last time, there was a feeling of "Now what? Where do I go from here?"

Write down the names of drugs YOU might be taking.

DO YOU NEED CHEMOTHERAPY?

That is the burning question on many women's minds. The recommendation to have chemotherapy will be made by your team of physicians after a review of all the data, including tumor size, spread to lymph nodes, and results of any genomic testing. The decision will depend on the size, grade, hormone receptor status, and HER2 status; your age, health, and menopausal status; and any lymph node involvement. Most importantly, it will depend on the results of genomic testing.

Genomic testing has proven to be one of the most valuable recent advances in the "chemo-no chemo" decision.

Using a sample of the woman's tumor tissue, Oncotype DX, the 21-gene expression assay, predicts the *chance or recurrence within the next ten years*.

Women with a high score of 26-100 receive both hormone therapy and chemotherapy. Those with a low score of 0-10 typically only need hormone therapy. Until recently, women in the intermediate 11-25 score range were in the gray zone, making decisions difficult.

But early in 2018 one of the largest and most reliable studies demonstrated that for women in this score range, with hormone receptor (HR)-positive, HER2-negative, axillary lymph node–negative breast cancer, treatment with chemotherapy and hormone therapy after surgery is no more beneficial than treatment with hormone therapy alone. This means that thousands of women will be able to avoid chemotherapy, with all of its side effects, while still achieving excellent long-term outcomes.

The study highlights the value using gene analysis to help deliver "personalized medicine" or "precision medicine".

Chemotherapy may also be used before surgery. This *neo-adjuvant chemotherapy* is often used to shrink ("downstage') a tumor before it is removed. The rationale is that a smaller tumor opens more options for breast conserving surgery and improved cosmetic results.

Neo-adjuvant chemo may be recommended for HER2/neu positive, or for triple negative tumors (cancers that tested negative for all three: estrogen receptors, progesterone receptors, and HER2), larger than 5mm (about a quarter of an inch). Why? Because knowing whether the tumor can be destroyed by the chemo is a great predictor of recurrence for these very aggressive tumors.

And for ER/PR positive tumors, tumors that typically do not respond to chemotherapy, women may be treated with neo-endocrine therapy with tamoxifen to shrink the tumor before surgery and allow for better margins, negative nodes and breast preservation if desired by the patient. *Endocrine*, or *hormone therapy* is the subject of the next chapter.

Armed with all this information, you and your physicians will discuss whether which therapy is appropriate for you. It is a complex issue, and you need to participate in the decision process.

CHAPTER 8

HORMONE THERAPY

Cancer that is confined to the breast area can be treated effectively with surgery and radiation therapy. Cancer that has spread to areas beyond the breast is much more difficult to treat. PET/CT and bone scans may give an indication of whether the spread has actually occured. Unfortunately, it is not always possible to determine with certainty at the time of diagnosis whether the cancer has spread or not.

Because of this, many clinicians recommend treatment with adjuvant, or additional therapy such as chemotherapy or hormonal therapy, or both, whenever there is a reasonable chance that cancer cells have metastasized to other parts of the body. The reasoning is that while hormone therapy and chemotherapy may be unpleasant, cancer recurrences can be life-threatening. Therefore the benefits outweigh the side effects.

Estrogen fits into receptor sites and stimulates cell division

What is Hormone Therapy?

Chemotherapy uses cytotoxic drugs to kill cancer cells. By contrast, *hormone therapy*, also called *endocrine therapy*, uses medications that prevent cancer cells from growing by changing normal body processes. Hormones are natural chemicals produced by the body to regulate various functions such as blood sugar metabolism, bone growth, or milk production in the breasts. Hormones include such substances as adrenaline, insulin, and estrogen.

Certain types of breast cancers can grow only when there is a supply of the female hormones estrogen or progesterone. By treating the patient with chemicals that block, add or remove the action of estrogen or progesterone, it is possible to slow down, or even stop, the growth of these cancer cells. Perhaps more accurately, it should be called ***anti-hormone therapy*** instead of hormone therapy.

Also, do not confuse hormone therapy for treatment of breast cancer with hormone replacement therapy, or HRT, for management of hot flashes and other symptoms during menopause. Different drugs, different goals.

How Does (Anti-)Hormone Therapy Work?

Those cancers that need estrogen or progesterone to grow are made of cells equipped with hormone receptor sites scattered over their surface. These cancers are called estrogen or progesterone receptor positive, or ER- or PR-positive. Estrogen or progesterone molecules fit into the receptor sites like keys into locks, and stimulate the cells to divide. This makes the tumor grow faster.

Different hormone therapies work in one of several ways: by blocking the receptor sites, by eliminating receptor sites entirely, or by decreasing hormone production.

Hormonal agents block estrogen binding sites

Blocking receptor sites: Tamoxifen and toremifene (Fareston)
These drugs, taken as daily pills, work by temporarily clogging the estrogen receptors site on the surface of the cancer cells, preventing estrogen molecules from binding to the cell. Think of it as the wrong key in a door lock: it fits, but won't turn, and keeps out the right key. The result: the cells are not stimulated, and the tumor stops growing.

In women whose cancers are ER- or PR-positive, treatment with tamoxifen for five years reduces breast cancer recurrence by half. Tamoxifen has also been shown to be effective in reducing the development of breast cancer in those women who are at high risk for the disease.

Eliminating hormone receptor sites: Fulvestrant (Faslodex)
Faslodex works by eliminating the hormone receptors on the surface of the cells, making the cells insensitive to the growth-enhancing effect of hormones. Faslodex is given by injection, once a month. It is approved for use only in postmenopausal women who do not respond to tamoxifen or Fareston.

Decreasing estrogen production: Aromatase inhibitors, or AI's
Aromatase is a natural enzyme that helps produce small but significant amounts of estrogen in postmenopausal women. Inhibiting this enzyme can be an effective way of preventing the body from producing hormones in the first place.

The currently approved aromatase inhibitors are letrozole (Femara), anastrozole (Arimidex) and exemestane (Aromasin). These drugs are not able to shut down estrogen production in women with fully functioning ovaries, so they are only used in postmenopausal women.

Whether alone or in combination with tamoxifen, aromatase inhibitors have been shown to reduce the risk of breast cancer recurrence better than tamoxifen alone.

Decreasing estrogen production: Ovarian ablation
Premenopausal women, whose ovaries are a major source of estrogen and progesterone, have more limited choices of hormone therapy. By eliminating the ovaries surgically (by a procedure called *oophorectomy*) or chemically (with drugs such as Zoladex) the women effectively become postmenopausal, and can take advantage of a wider variety of hormone treatment options.

VICKI

Tamoxifen made sense. The only side effect I've had is some hot flashes, and the vaginal dryness. I use a vaginal ring that releases a tiny amount of estrogen, just locally. My gynecologist said that is safe. And it does help.

QUESTIONS TO ASK
YOUR DOCTOR:

What side effects should I expect?

Can I get pregnant while taking tamoxifen?

What birth control method would be most suitable to my lifestyle?

Side Effects of Hormone Therapy

The side effects of hormone therapy vary with the type of therapy used. In general, hormone therapy has far fewer, and less severe, side effects than chemotherapy. Because hormone therapy blocks estrogen, it may cause the same symptoms as going through menopause, including hot flashes, changes in menstrual periods and vaginal dryness.

Hormone therapy may affect the rate of loss of calcium from bones, which may lead to osteoporosis. Ask your physician if you need a *bone density test* to determine whether your bones are in danger of becoming too brittle.

While you are on hormone therapy, you may still get pregnant, even if your periods have stopped as a result of the treatment. Since hormone therapy may be harmful to the fetus, it's important to use birth control if you are sexually active. Do not use an oral contraceptive, or an injection or implant that contains hormones, since they may interfere with your hormone therapy. Instead, use a barrier method, such as a condom or a diaphragm.

Feel free to discuss with your doctor or nurse any sexual difficulties that you may be experiencing due to hormone therapy. Remember, there are many ways of helping you maintain your sexual activity even while you are being treated. In Chapter 13 we will review the sexual side effects of cancer therapy in greater detail.

Weight Gain

Even though you are being treated for cancer, your weight may increase, rather than decrease, sometimes by as much as 10-20 lbs. Many women find this side effect distressing.

Who Should be Treated With Hormone Therapy?

Not all types of breast cancer can be treated with hormone therapy. If your tumor is estrogen receptor positive (ER+) or progesterone receptor positive (PR+), it means that the tumor can be stimulated by these hormones. In this case, your medical oncologist may recommend hormone therapy. If the tests are negative, hormone therapy will have no effect on the growth of your cancer.

CHAPTER 9

TARGETED THERAPY

What Are Targeted Therapies?

Chemotherapy drugs work by attacking all fast-growing cells in the body. Fortunately, this includes cancer cells. Unfortunately, it also includes the rapidly multiplying but normal cells of the gastrointestinal tract, bone marrow, skin, and other organs.

For a long time, scientists have been looking for new drugs that could tell the difference between normal and cancerous cells. The search has produced results.

Targeted therapy, also called *immunotherapy* or *biological therapy*, is a promising approach to cancer treatment that is designed to target cancer cells specifically. It works differently from cell-killing chemotherapy and has different side effects.

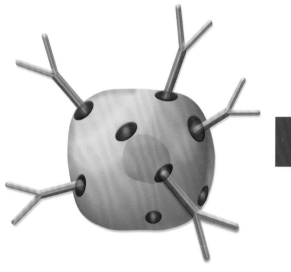

Target therapy molecules home in on specific receptor sites on the surface of a breast cancer cell

Herceptin (trastuzumab) and others

The first targeted therapy compound to gain acceptance in breast cancer treatment was Herceptin, a *monoclonal antibody*.

What exactly is a monoclonal antibody? An *antibody* is a protein naturally produced by the body to fight off all foreign particles. A *monoclonal* antibody is a protein created in a laboratory, and tailor-made to target very specific "foreign particles": certain cancer cells.

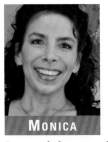

I persuaded my oncologist to give me smaller doses of the drug for longer periods of time, so my side effects were almost not noticeable. Just make sure that this kind of regimen is the right thing for you.

To manufacture a monoclonal antibody, tumor cells from the patient are inactivated and then injected into a laboratory animal to stimulate the production of antibodies specific to that cancer. When the antibodies are removed and injected into the patient, they bypass healthy tissues, and home-in directly on the tumor cells.

Herceptin is engineered to interfere with a growth-promoting protein known as HER2/neu. This protein is present in abnormally high amounts on the surface of breast cancer cells in about one out of five breast cancer patients.

So Herceptin is used as an adjuvant treatment of HER2 overexpressing, node-positive or node-negative (ER/PR negative or with one high risk feature breast cancer) as part of a regimen consisting of one or several drugs, or as a single agent.

It is also used with paclitaxel for first-line treatment of HER2-overexpressing metastatic breast cancer or as a single agent for treatment of HER2-overexpressing breast cancer in patients who have received one or more chemotherapy regimens for metastatic disease.

Herceptin and other monoclonal antibodies are not free of side effects. These may include a wide variety of symptoms such as fever and chills, weakness, nausea, vomiting, cough, diarrhea, headache.

Avastin (bevacizumab)

Drugs Herceptin and Tykerb are designed to attack cancer cells that are rich in HER2 protein. Avastin has a different action. In fact, it is not considered a "targeted therapy." Instead, it works by blocking the growth of new blood vessels that supply nutrients to cancer cells. Deprived of nutrients, the tumor dies, or at least fails to grow and spread.

Avastin was at one point approved for the treatment of patients with metastatic HER2-negative breast cancer. But then the FDA announced that it had removed the breast cancer indication from Avastin because the drug has not been shown to be safe and effective for that use. The medicine itself is not being removed from the market and doctors can choose to use Avastin to treat metastatic breast cancer whether or not that particular use is officially approved by the FDA.

Who Can Benefit From Targeted Therapy?
A sample of your tumor will be sent for a variety of tests, either right after the biopsy, or at a later date, to determine which, if any, targeted therapies could benefit you. Your physician is the only one who can advise you about the risks and expected benefits in your particular case.

THE FUTURE

Scientists are searching for new markers that will help them develop additional, and better-focused, targeted therapies. Ask your doctor to review the latest findings with you.

Many experts believe that new technologies may bring new hope for effective treatment, cure, or even prevention of breast cancer.

QUESTIONS TO ASK YOUR DOCTOR:

Is targeted therapy right for me?

Would I benefit more from chemotherapy, hormonal therapy or targeted therapy?

How will I know if Herceptin is helping me?

Are there any clinical trials that I qualify for?

CHAPTER 10

COMPLEMENTARY AND ALTERNATIVE THERAPIES

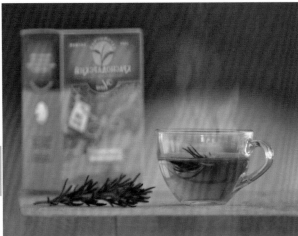

You will probably hear about things like acupuncture, antioxidants, macrobiotic diets, imagery, aromatherapy, as well as other "complementary" or "alternative therapies". It's extremely important that you understand the difference between conventional medicine, and complementary or alternative therapies.

Conventional treatment is what is currently accepted by reputable healthcare providers. It is based on decades of sound medical research, and represents the best that Western medicine has to offer today.

Complementary treatments may or may not have been evaluated as rigorously as conventional treatment, but they are widely and successfully used to relieve side effects of cancer treatment, and to enhance the quality of life.

Alternative therapies, by contrast, have no medically sound foundation, and no credible evidence of any beneficial effect. They represent a dangerous temptation for those who may be skeptical about traditional medical treatment.

Consult your healthcare team before trying any type of complementary therapy to make sure it won't interfere with your treatment. And certainly have an informed discussion with them if you are contemplating embarking on an alternative course of treatment. Your health and even your life are at stake.

COMPLEMENTARY THERAPIES

Practitioners refer to these therapies as *complementary*, rather than *alternative*, because they are to be used only in conjunction with—not instead of—the treatment recommended by your doctors. You still need surgery, or chemotherapy or whatever other conventional treatment is right for you.

There is a wide variety of complementary techniques, some based on principles adopted from other specialties (for example, relaxation), from Oriental medicine (acupuncture) from Indian medicine (yoga), or even from ancient Egyptian culture (aromatherapy).

Mind/Body Connection

Many complementary therapies are based on the principle of *mind/body connection*. For centuries, people have believed that there is a connection between the state of the mind and the health of the body. How this connection worked, however, was never quite clear.

Recently, scientists have identified chemicals, called *neurotransmitters*, by which nerve cells communicate with one another. Neurotransmitters are also involved in the control of emotions. For example, antidepressant medications increase the amount of norepinephrine and serotonin in the spaces between nerve cells. These same neurotransmitters have effects elsewhere in the body, affecting heart rate and blood pressure, and may even influence the activity of cells in the immune system.

Changes in the state of the nervous system which can occur because of stress or lack of social support, can influence many organ systems. For example, it has been found that people under stress are more likely to develop colds.

Anxiety, grief, stress, and fear of the unknown all seem to have an impact on the body. Learning to cope with these emotions, using a wide variety of approaches—such as meditation and visualization, spiritual support, and participation in support groups—may help speed your recovery, and benefit your health.

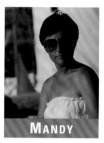

MANDY

I listened to tapes by Bernie Siegel, read motivational literature and practical self-hypnosis books. I took vitamins, especially C, E, and beta carotene. I rode my exercise bike almost daily. When I felt weak, I napped and tried not to feel guilty about sleeping during the day. I believe all these therapies were an important part of my recovery.

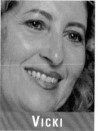

VICKI

I started seeing an acupuncturist early on during the treatment. I was very careful to check it with my oncologist first, to make sure it wasn't going to affect my treatment. The goal was to keep my energy up and my nausea down. So I never threw up from the chemo.

Meditation and Visualization

Many healthcare professionals refer to "meditation" and "visualization" as "stress reduction," or "relaxation."

Meditation has been shown to produce physiological responses such as a decrease in blood pressure, respiration rate, and overall metabolism—all of which contribute to reducing stress on our minds and bodies. Guided imagery or visualization (for example, visualizing natural killer cells gobbling up cancers cells like in the old game Pac-Man) can also be used with meditation.

There is no claim that meditation and visualization can cure cancer, but studies have proven that a combination of these techniques can reduce pain and other uncomfortable side effects of cancer treatment.

Spiritual Support

Since prehistoric times, prayer has been one of the most common ways of dealing with pain and illness in all civilizations. Today many accept that some form of spiritual support is a basic human need. Prayer, laying on of hands, and many forms of spiritual imagery or inner dialogue have helped patients find the higher strength within themselves to cope with breast cancer and other illness.

Many cancer patients rely on their religious traditions to regain control and gather additional strength to battle cancer. Even those who have little or no connection with religion, often find themselves moved by the "spiritual emergency" of cancer.

Humor / Laughter

Laughter can stimulate endorphins—chemicals that act like opiates in the brain. You might find humor and laughter emotionally healing. In addition, giving yourself time not to think about your cancer can have a wonderfully invigorating effect.

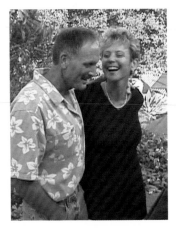

When undergoing cancer treatment, writer Norman Cousins discovered that ten minutes of genuine belly laughter had an anesthetic effect that would give him at least two hours of pain-free sleep.

Diet

There's still a great deal of controversy on the subject of nutrition and its effect on breast cancer. So far, there's no scientific data to prove one diet is better than another for breast cancer treatment.

Most physicians recommend that patients simply follow good nutrition, with particular emphasis on protein and vitamins during chemotherapy treatment. A consultation with a nutritionist will help you learn more about your particular needs.

Macrobiotic diets emphasize whole grains, miso soup, fresh vegetables and beans, with little fruit and no sugar. Special diets such as these may some-day prove to be effective for patients with certain types of cancer, but more scientific research is needed in this area.

Herbal Therapy

The majority of herbal therapies are based on the belief that they improve organ function. There is increasing evidence from Asian and European countries that some herbs can be effective in fighting cancer. Common herbs and medicinal plants used for breast cancer include Astragalus root, burdock root, garlic, green tea, licorice root and a variety of others.

Some herbal preparations are extremely potent and may be harmful. You should always consult your healthcare professional before beginning herbal therapy, since some preparations may interfere with your treatment.

Vitamins

Many biological processes in the body lead to the formation of toxic products such as toxic lipid peroxides, which can damage DNA in cells, leading to cancer. Vitamins C, E, and beta-carotene are "antioxidant" vitamins commonly used to neutralize these potentially toxic products. In addition, elements such as selenium and copper may be useful, in trace amounts only, to facilitate the defense against toxic peroxides.

Antioxidants may interfere with the beneficial effects of radiation, and should be used only with the approval of your radiation oncologist. Contact the National Cancer Institute or the American Cancer Society to find out about the latest recommendations on the topic of antioxidants and vitamins.

BETSY

I got back into meditation, into bio-feedback, into guided imagery. I cleaned up my diet, took the vitamins that I needed to take, and the herbs, and looked into acupuncture and some other modalities. And I think it really enhanced the way I dealt with chemo. I never threw up. I never lost all of my hair, though I was told that I would.

Acupuncture

Acupuncture and homeopathy are based on the concept that there is a *life force* within our body organs. This life force maintains the body in a state of health, but predisposes us to disease when it is unbalanced.

Acupuncture is a technique, first developed in ancient China, which involves insertion of needles at specific points in the body to balance the life force.

The theory behind acupuncture is that there are special meridian points on the body that are connected to internal organs. Vital energy flows along the meridian lines, and diseases are caused by an imbalance of this flow. Normal flow of vital energy is restored by inserting needles at the meridian points.

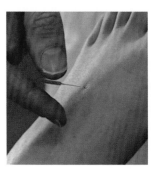

Current research suggests that acupuncture needles may work by triggering the release of natural pain inhibitors.

In China, acupuncture has long been used for pain relief, and for treatment of ailments such as arthritis, hypertension, and ulcers. A growing number of Western physicians use acupuncture to relieve nausea, pain or other symptoms associated with cancer.

Homeopathy

Practitioners of homeopathy believe that minute, highly diluted doses of a medicine treat the life force of organs such as the liver, kidneys, or intestines. Although homeopathy is questioned by most American physicians, it is widely used in Europe and Asia.

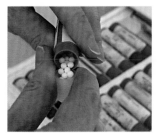

ALTERNATIVE TREATMENTS

Alternative treatments are treatments that are used *instead of* standard medical care. They can be dangerous in several ways: by depriving you of potentially life-saving conventional treatment, or by leading you to use substances that are in themselves harmful to your body.

It takes years of painstaking work to develop a treatment for cancer, and more years to prove beyond a doubt that it is effective and safe. From time to time, a new product suddenly appears, and is promoted as the new miracle cure, and an appealing alternative to standard medical treatment. Be very careful. Most of the time, the claims are founded on a few poorly documented cases of alleged "cures," and sometimes on nothing but a promoter's greed or ignorance.

If you are considering an alternative therapy, make sure to balance promotional information provided by sellers with objective, evidence-based information that you can obtain from your healthcare provider.

QUESTIONS TO ASK:

What benefits can be expected from this therapy?

What are the risks associated with this therapy?

Do the known benefits outweigh the risks?

What side effects can be expected?

Will the therapy interfere with conventional treatment?

Will the therapy be covered by health insurance?

Tips for Evaluating Alternative Therapy Claims

- The product is advertised as a quick and effective cure-all.

- The promoters use words like "scientific breakthrough", "miraculous cure", "exclusive product", "secret ingredient" or "ancient remedy".

- The promoter claims the government, the medical profession or research scientists have conspired to suppress the product.

- The advertisement includes results that are "amazing" but undocumented.

- The product is advertised as available from only one source, and payment is required in advance.

- The promoter promises a no-risk "money-back guarantee." Many won't be around to respond to your request for a refund.

NINA-Nurse Navigator

If you are still adamant about using an alternative treatment, please consider using the conventional therapy alongside it. After all, it can only increase your chances of a cure, not decrease them!

CHAPTER 11

DCIS

This chapter deals with DCIS—*ductal carcinoma in situ*—a very early, non-invasive breast cancer, classified as Stage 0. If you were diagnosed with a higher stage of cancer, you may skip this chapter.

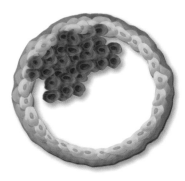

In situ cancer. Cancer cells have not penetrated through the membrane of the duct

What is DCIS?

DCIS is a ductal cancer that has not yet penetrated the lining of the duct. In other words, it is not invasive. In this in situ ("in place") stage, the cancer has not spread into the blood stream and beyond. If it is diagnosed and treated correctly, the risk of dying from this cancer is essentially zero.

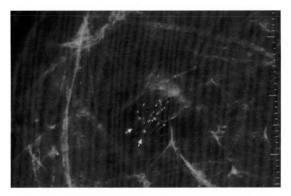

Microcalcifications of DCIS appear as tiny white dots on a digital mammogram

In the past, DCIS was rare—most breast cancers were found when the tumor had grown large enough to be felt by hand. By then it had time to spread outside the breast. But with the increased use of mammography, DCIS has become relatively easy to detect. It appears on mammograms as *microcalcifications*: a speckling of tiny white dots that are clumps of dead cancer cells that became calcified inside the ducts.

Ductal carcinoma in situ is the most common type of non-invasive breast cancer. DCIS has not yet been researched as extensively as the more common invasive breast cancer, and there is some disagreement among physicians as to how to treat it.

Mastectomy or Lumpectomy?

Until recently, it was firmly believed that the best way to treat DCIS was to perform a simple mastectomy. The feeling was that since the cancer has not yet spread (remember, DCIS is in situ!) all one had to do was remove the breast for essentially a 100% guarantee of cure. No chemotherapy, no radiation, no lymph node dissection.

When lumpectomy plus radiation became an acceptable choice for invasive breast cancer, surgeons learned that if they removed a small DCIS tumor with a wide margin around it, and treated the breast with radiation, they could achieve a much nicer cosmetic result.

But lumpectomy does carry a small chance of future local cancer recurrence. So the choice of treatment—mastectomy or lumpectomy—is up to the patient, and depends on her ability to tolerate a risk that is a little higher than zero.

Radiation Therapy or Not?

The other area where there may be a difference of opinion is radiation therapy. A Stage I or II (invasive) tumor treated with breast conserving surgery will almost always be treated with radiation too. But some specialists believe that there is no need for irradiating the breast if the DCIS tumor was small, and the margins were large and clear—in other words, if there is a fair degree of certainty that the tumor was indeed in situ.

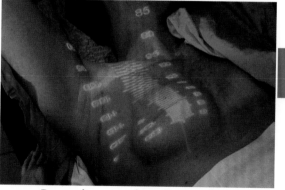

Beam alignment for radiation therapy

The reason to avoid radiation is that if the cancer does come back as an invasive cancer, the patient will no longer have the option of breast conserving surgery, since radiation therapy can be used only once on the same area. The next time, treatment will require a mastectomy, rather than a lumpectomy. This is another dilemma that requires discussion with your healthcare team.

QUESTIONS TO ASK:

What grade is my DCIS?

How well will I do without radiation?

Do you work with a team that includes a mammographer and an experienced pathologist?

What is the downside of getting radiation after surgical removal of the DCIS tumor?

TREATMENT OF DCIS

To make the decisions easier, researchers devised a system for selecting the best treatment plan for each DCIS lesion. It is based on the size of the tumor, the grade of the tumor cells, and the width of the margins around the tumor. Here is how the procedure runs:

Before surgery, an accurate mammogram is obtained, to determine exactly the size and shape of the DCIS lesion.

During the operation, the surgeon removes the tumor with a large margin of normal tissue, striving for at least a half inch on all sides.

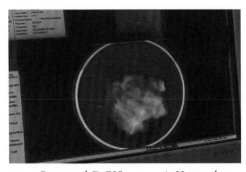

Removed DCIS tumor is X-rayed

The radiologist takes an X-ray of the tissue removed and compares it with the original mammogram, to ensure that the entire tumor was removed.

Immediately after the X-ray, while the patient is still in the operating room, a pathologist makes numerous slices across the tumor and examines each slice in detail. Applying black ink to the outside of the tumor makes it easier to determine if the margins are "clear."

If the tumor was small, the grade of the cells was low, and the margins were at least 10mm (less than half an inch) there may be no need for removing additional tissue, or for radiation therapy.

If the tumor was larger, the cells more aggressive, or the margins too narrow, then the DCIS tumor may be treated with a simple mastectomy, or lumpectomy with radiation.

Your Team

If you were diagnosed with DCIS, you may consider investing some time into finding a medical center with an experienced team—a surgeon, a pathologist and a mammographer who work well together in assessing in situ tumors. In this way you will be assured of the best chances for a successful treatment, with the least loss of breast tissue.

CHAPTER 12

CLINICAL TRIALS

WHAT ARE TRIALS?

Scientists are constantly searching for better ways of dealing with breast cancer. Many women diagnosed with breast cancer may benefit from this research by participating in clinical trials.

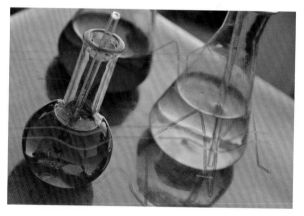

A clinical trial is an evaluation of a new way of managing cancer. Some trials are designed to see if a new drug or a new procedure will be more effective in treating or preventing cancer than the existing method. Other trials evaluate new ways to diagnose the disease. Still others concentrate on finding a new way to eliminate unwanted side effects.

Clinical trials help improve the quality of care, now and in the future. One such trial, conducted many years ago, showed that lumpectomy with radiation treatment was as effective as removal of the entire breast, which was the standard practice back then. As a result of this trial, many women today can enjoy the benefits of breast-conserving surgery.

Clinical trials are not random attempts to discover something new. Trials are conducted according to very specific guidelines that are recognized by the medical community worldwide. By ensuring uniformity, it is possible to be confident that results obtained in one location, will be readily comparable to results from another location, even in another country.

When the word "research" was first presented to me, I felt very fearful: Is this something that's only been tried on me? Am I the research rat? But when I learned more, I realized that it wasn't like that. I felt very fortunate knowing that I was getting aggressive therapy and that I would only benefit from it.

QUESTIONS TO ASK ABOUT A CLINICAL TRIAL:

How do I know the facility doing the study is reputable?

Are there other centers doing the same research on the same drugs or methods?

What is involved in terms of tests, treatments, and additional time commitments?

What results can be reasonably expected in my particular case?

New treatments are first tested in laboratories, using animals. Animal research offers scientists the only way to make the transition from something that works in a test tube to something that will work in people, without risking human lives unnecessarily in the process.

If there is initial evidence that the treatment may be effective, it is then evaluated further with actual patients, usually with advanced stages of the disease.

To reach the next trial stage, where large numbers of patients are used, the treatment method or drug must have demonstrated that it offers potential benefit, without unacceptable risk.

If the clinical trial confirms the benefits, the drug or treatment will be made available to all patients.

HOW ARE TRIALS CONDUCTED?

Every trial is conducted according to a protocol—a set of guidelines that spells out exactly what will be done and when. Large numbers of patients are selected according to very specific criteria—age, stage of cancer, previous treatment, and so forth.

The patients who meet these criteria are enrolled into the study, and divided into groups. Most trials consist of a control group (patients who are receiving standard therapy) and a treatment group (those who receive the new therapy that is being evaluated.) The treatment group always receives treatment that is considered to be at least as good, and possibly better, than the standard treatment. Sometimes the control group receives a placebo— an injection or a pill that looks like the drug being evaluated, but has no medicinal value; for example, a sugar pill instead of a drug.

Patients are assigned to one of the two groups by a random, computerized system, where neither the patient nor the physician has control over the selection. In addition, neither the patient nor the investigator knows which group the patient was placed in, until the end of the trial. This process is called double-blind randomization. The purpose of double-blind randomization is to avoid bias on the part of the patient and of the treating physician. Not knowing whether the actual drug or a placebo is being administered eliminates preconceived notions. This keeps the patient from reporting improvement or side effects that may be imaginary. And it keeps the researcher from favoring one or the other group, and skewing the results.

A central agency keeps all the records of the random selection, and can reveal them if the need arises. For example, if one group is showing a significantly better response than the other, the trial is terminated, and all patients are given the better treatment.

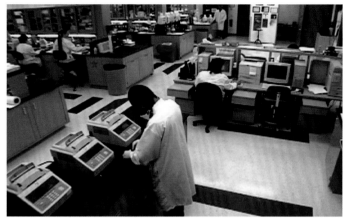

New drugs must pass extensive testing before being approved

PARTICIPATING IN A TRIAL

If your physician does not mention trials, bring up the subject on your own. There are many trials going on around the country, and you may find one that matches your case perfectly. There is information about ongoing trials on the National Cancer Institute's hotline called PDQ, or from the local chapter of the American Cancer Society.

You and your physician will review the lists of requirements for various trials to see whether or not you might qualify for one of them. If you do, be sure to find out what is involved in terms of tests, treatments, additional time commitments, and side effects, and evaluate whether or not you can live with these terms for an extended time. Then assess the possible benefits to you, and balance them against the negatives.

If you decide to proceed, you will be asked to sign an informed consent form, to show that you understand the issues involved, the expected benefits, the possible side effects, your rights and responsibilities, and the possible outcome.

You will be asked to follow the schedule of treatments and tests as closely as possible, in order to make the information obtained scientifically sound.

QUESTIONS TO ASK ABOUT A CLINICAL TRIAL:

What are the currently accepted treatments and how do they compare to the trial?

How can I be sure that I won't be under-treated, or miss the opportunity to be treated with established, conventional therapy?

What would my financial commitment be and how can I cope with it?

Will I need to be available for follow-up testing indefinitely?

Can I travel, work, or move to another city?

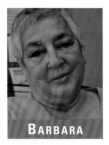

BARBARA

When I was asked to be on a
research study, it was very
carefully explained to me by
my doctor and his nurse.
I took a copy of the papers
home, and as a matter of
fact, sent one to a female
physician friend of mine. We
talked on the phone about it.
I felt that I would be carefully watched and carefully
monitored. So I had no hesi-
tation.

IS A TRIAL RIGHT FOR ME?

Trials are what makes it possible for medicine to make progress. But you
won't be participating purely for the good of others. Being part of a trial
offers a definite benefit for you personally, whether you are assigned to the
treatment group and receive the new drug, or you are enrolled in the control group and receive conventional therapy.

One of the advantages of being in a clinical trial is that patients in both treatment and control groups enjoy a higher standard of care, because trial pro-
tocols usually call for more frequent tests, more frequent visits to the hospital, and more thorough examinations.

And there are few, if any, downsides. Your participation is completely
optional and voluntary. You can leave the trial at any time. If you drop out,
you will not be penalized in any way, and you will still be entitled to the best
standard treatment available.

CHAPTER 13

LIFE AFTER CANCER

You had your last dose of chemotherapy, or your last radiation treatment. The surgical scars are beginning to heal. As your energy and confidence return, you'll be able to explore the many options for moving forward from the cancer experience, to a new life.

EMOTIONAL RECOVERY

A diagnosis of cancer impacts your self-esteem, your body image, your sexuality—even your outlook on survival. You probably realize that life will never be the same after such an experience. This will leave you with a sense of loss. Take time to grieve the loss. This grieving process is an important first step toward the healing of the mind.

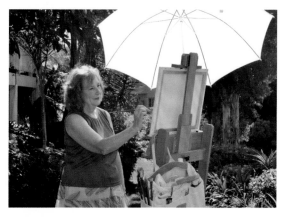

Do something you've always wanted to do!

Reactive Depression

As you try to come to terms with your diagnosis and try to deal with the impact of your treatment, you are likely to have episodes of anxiety and depression. It is important for you to distinguish depression that you can cope with on your own, from depression that requires professional help.

As is the case for most women undergoing cancer treatment, there will be times when you are sad—times when you are "feeling blue". This is called *reactive depression*—in other words, you are having an appropriate reaction to your situation. This level of depression is normal, and most women can cope with it, with help from family, friends, or support groups.

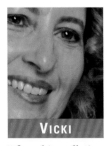

VICKI

I found it really important to stay busy. It keeps you from sitting there and thinking that life is passing by. Creating my website has been a wonderful, uplifting experience.

QUESTIONS TO ASK YOUR
DOCTOR OR NURSE:

What can I do if I wake up at night worrying about my cancer?

Shouldn't we be doing more testing on me to make sure the cancer didn't come back?

Why have I lost interest in intimate relations with my partner?

Why can't I sleep or relax or feel interested in anything?

One method that helps manage anxiety and depression is planning pleasant activities such as going out with friends or seeing a movie around the times when you normally feel depressed.

Another approach is exercise and sports. Physical activity stimulates the body to produce certain chemicals called endorphins that help restore a sense of well being. Try to get out of your mind and into your body, so to speak.

Other effective techniques include relaxation and visualization, described in the chapter on Complementary Therapies.

If you haven't already, consider joining a support group. You should have no trouble finding one that matches your lifestyle and your particular needs.

There are specific times during the course of treatment and recovery when bouts of anxiety and depression are more likely to occur. Most women experience their highest level of anxiety when they come home from the hospital after surgery, because coming home means leaving most of the medical team behind and resuming normal activities.

Another time women may feel anxious or depressed is when their chemotherapy or radiation treatments end. There may be a feeling of panic at the thought that you are not being treated any more. This post-treatment anxiety is quite natural, and will gradually diminish as you regain confidence.

Some women notice that they are particularly anxious on the anniversary dates of their diagnosis or surgery. These are the so-called anniversary reactions. In addition, many women also may have "checkup anxiety" just before their scheduled follow-up visit to the physician.

Clinical Depression

There is a form of depression that is unlikely to improve on its own. Usually it includes continuous feelings of sadness, feelings of worthlessness or guilt, excessive fear of the future, and lack of interest in intimacy or sex. This is called clinical depression and requires intervention by a trained professional.

Clinical depression can be treated. It may involve counseling, medications, and perhaps physical exercise and stress reduction techniques. Your physician will be able to refer you to the appropriate specialist.

And remember, you should never feel embarrassed to seek professional help. It is not a sign of weakness—no more so than going to a surgeon for a lumpectomy. Most cases of depression are short, and usually respond to counseling, with or without the use of some of the very effective medications available today.

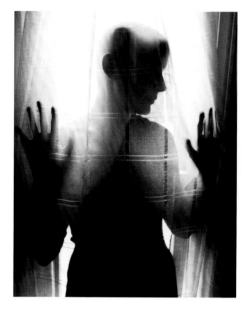

Trapped by clinical depression

If you experience several of these symptoms, you should discuss your situation with your physician. If you have thoughts about suicide, call your physician or nurse immediately.

You may have a clinical depression if you:

- Are continuously sad for weeks
- Withdraw from friends and relatives
- Feel worthless
- Fear the future excessively
- Speak or move slowly
- Feel tired all the time
- Can't make decisions
- Are angry all the time
- Lost interest in intimacy and sex

PHYSICAL RECOVERY

Ask your nurse navigator to give you a survivorship plan. This form will summarize your treatment, your team and the recommended follow-up.

Regular Follow-Up

Even after the most complete treatment, there's always a chance that cancer will recur. Most recurrences happen two or three years after surgery. The longer you go without a recurrence, the greater are your chances of remaining free of disease. But you can never say that the cancer has been completely cured.

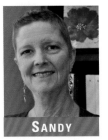

SANDY

When I walked out of the chemo suite for the last time, there was a feeling of, "Now what? Where do I go from here?" I wasn't treating my cancer anymore. But I got over it. I still get a little tense when I go for my checkups.

Because of this possibility, you need regular follow-up visits with a healthcare professional. It could be your family physician, your oncologist, or your breast surgeon. What's important is to have a single person in charge of the follow-up care. Usually you'll be seen as often as every few weeks immediately after treatment, and perhaps only every six months later on. There is no "right" schedule. Eventually, you will probably be down to a single annual visit.

What does follow-up involve? Most physicians suggest a physical examination to look for signs of local recurrence—new lumps within the breast after lumpectomy, or tiny hard nodules in the surgical scar after mastectomy.

In addition, mammography will be scheduled on a regular basis, and you may have a number of blood tests that will assess the function of your liver, bone marrow, and other organs, and a chest X-ray. Other tests such as CEA (carcinoembryonic antigen, a protein found in the blood of patients with cancer) and bone scans are not used routinely.

Currently, many experts feel that there is little to be gained by performing multiple tests on patients that are asymptomatic—that is patients who have no symptoms. Such tests may detect a recurrence a few months earlier, but earlier diagnosis will not change the outcome of whatever treatment you might need. So you can expect to have fewer and fewer tests as the years pass after your initial treatment.

Breast Self-Examination (BSE)

BSE is particularly important for women at higher risk of breast cancer—and that includes you and your first degree relatives. You need to become familiar with the new look and feel of your breasts, so that you can report any changes promptly.

BSE is not a skill that you can learn from a brochure or a shower card. The best way to learn it is from your healthcare provider, or from a good breast self-exam DVD or online video, such as offered by the Susan G. Komen Foundation.

A thorough BSE should include:

Looking. Using a mirror, check the shape and size of your breasts, and the color and texture of your skin, first with your arms down, then with your arms in the air. Try to learn what's normal for you, so that you can spot any changes immediately.

Feeling. Lie down with a folded towel under your shoulder. Extend the arm out at an angle to spread the breast tissue more evenly.

Use three middle fingers to examine the entire breast area. Make three dime-sized circles. One just lightly, one deeper, one deeper still. This will enable you to check the full thickness of your breast. When you've finished, lower your arm and examine your armpit for possible lymph node enlargement.

If you had a mastectomy you are not likely to find a lump within the flap tissue used for reconstruction. Local recurrences are more likely to appear as tiny firm beads along the incision line.

If you had a lumpectomy, you will probably feel irregular lumpiness at the surgical sight shortly after the lumpectomy heals.

Clinical Breast Examination (CBE)

CBE will be part of your regular check ups. The physician will probably spend additional time examining the scar and areas where enlarged lymph nodes may be found—under the arms, and around the collar bones.

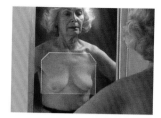

*Check your breasts
in the mirror*

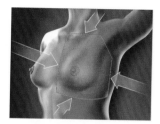

*Examine the entire
breast area*

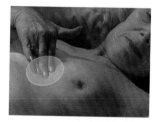

*Make three little circles
with your fingertips*

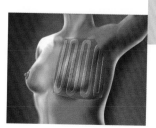

*Move your fingers
in vertical strips*

Mammography

Every woman who has had breast cancer should have a mammogram once a year, regardless of age.

If you had a lumpectomy, the films may be more difficult to interpret, so make sure that previous mammograms are available for comparison. If you had a mastectomy, you should have mammograms of the other breast.

If you are sensitive near the post-surgical scar, ask the technologist for special padding that fits on the mammography device.

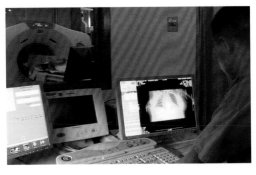

MRI

For women with especially dense breasts, or women who present unusual diagnostic challenges, MRI is an effective option.

In fact, the American Cancer Society now recommends that all women at high risk of breast cancer (which includes women who already had breast cancer before) should have screening with MRI every year.

Care of the Surgical Arm

After a mastectomy and particularly if you also had a lymph node dissection, your arm may feel numb and tingly due to nerve damage during surgery. Later, you may feel shooting pains due to nerve re-growth. There is not much that you can do to reverse numbness due to nerve damage. Some of it may improve as the nerves heal over the years.

NINA-Nurse Navigator

You may also need other studies besides mammography, like MRI or ultrasound. Just because the first cancer was found on mammo, doesn't mean another will show up the same way. Be alert!

Your healthcare professional will tell you which exercises are appropriate to help your arm regain its mobility and strength.

A more serious condition to watch for is lymphedema—swelling of the arm due to scarring of the lymph ducts after axillary surgery. The first signs might be subtle: tightness in your rings and clothes, and a feeling of fullness when you make a fist. It is important that you always follow your medical team's recommendations about how to avoid injury to the arm to reduce the chances of developing lymphedema.

INTIMACY AND SEXUALITY

Your Self-Image

We live in a society that considers breasts to be an important aspect of a woman's attractiveness. The loss of a breast after a mastectomy, or even a slight change in shape after a lumpectomy may have a serious impact on a woman's confidence. "Will I still be loved?" "Will I be attractive?" are valid questions that need to be answered in a woman's mind.

Doubts about your appearance and attractiveness are normal, but you should not let them affect your self-image. Remember, there is much more to sexuality and pleasure—and to you as a person—than the shape or presence of a breast.

The critical issue is not the loss of the breast itself, but the way you and your partner treat the loss. Open communication is very important. Many couples find to their surprise that the patient is more concerned about the loss of her breast than her partner is. The partner is often relieved that you are alive and will be getting well.

Side Effects of Treatment

The side effects of treatment will vary with the treatment choice, and with your own response.

Many of the side effects are easy to anticipate. Surgery could decrease or eliminate entirely nipple sensation—which may affect sexual arousal. Radiation therapy may render breast skin more irritable during treatment, and perhaps less sensitive years later. Overall, the emotional and physical demands of treatment take their toll, leading to fatigue. Most of these side effects are relatively short lived, or tolerable.

Other consequences of treatment may have a greater impact. For example, if you did not yet go through menopause, chemotherapy or hormonal therapy is almost certain to stop your periods—temporarily or permanently. If you are young, your periods are more likely to return than if you are approaching menopause.

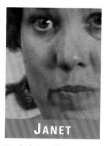

JANET

It didn't affect my sexual relationship at all. Maybe it enlightened it because I think that our love grew from the experience. It definitely didn't get worse.

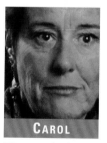

CAROL

The sexual relationships that I was in after the mastectomy required communication that hadn't been there before. I had to be able to tell people what would feel good.

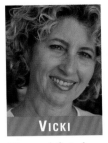

VICKI

Chemo definitely made sex more challenging. Fatigue, loss of libido, vaginal dryness... But my husband and I found ways to take care of these problems.

Menopause caused by chemotherapy is much more sudden, and for many women, more difficult than natural menopause. You may find that you are having mood swings that are out of character for you, and blame them on your inability to deal with cancer, whereas in reality you may be the victim of severe hormonal imbalance induced by the chemotherapy or hormone therapy.

Discuss your problems with your physician. Drugs like Celexa, Paxil, Prozac and others have proven very useful in dealing with menopausal symptoms.

A less recognized side effect is that chemotherapy reduces the amounts of testosterone in the body. Testosterone is generally known only as a male hormone, but it is present in small quantities in women, and is responsible for the woman's sex drive. With loss of testosterone, there is loss of libido—a side effect that often goes unnoticed, unreported, misdiagnosed, or untreated. If loss of libido becomes a problem for you and your partner, you may want to find a healthcare provider who is well versed in the management of such problems.

FERTILITY

Even in couples who have not yet had children, the urgency of dealing with breast cancer often takes precedence over plans to build a family. Sometimes rash treatment decisions are made that cannot later be reversed. For example, embarking on a course of hormone therapy or chemotherapy may lead to infertility that is not reversible. For younger couples, future fertility is one area that merits as much research as any other aspect of breast cancer treatment.

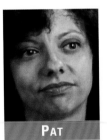

PAT

I would like to have children. Two doctors have said "No," and one has said it's OK. So, we're in limbo right now. If the hormone receptors were negative, there would be no problem with getting pregnant.

Breast cancer in itself does not rule out the possibility of having children. Many women go on to have successful pregnancies, with no adverse effect on their health or future outcome. If you're in your childbearing years and would like to have a baby, it is very important to discuss this issue with all the physicians on your team, including your oncologist, radiation therapist, pathologist, and surgeon. Ask them to review all the details of your case—such as cancer type, degree of spread, amount of radiation you received, and so on—before advising you on whether it is safe for you to get pregnant.

Recent advances in fertility offer new options for women who must undergo treatment that is likely to destroy the eggs in their ovaries and render them sterile.

One option is embryo freezing. For this procedure a few of the woman's eggs are surgically removed, artificially fertilized in vitro then frozen and stored for future re-implantation in the woman's uterus. This procedure has a 10-25% success rate.

Another option is removal and storage of unfertilized eggs—a good option if the woman is not in a relationship. This procedure has a lower (3%) success rate. Make sure you review all your options with a fertility expert.

RESUMING SEXUAL ACTIVITY

Some women and many of their partners worry about when and how it is acceptable to resume sexual activity after breast surgery. Sometimes the partner may avoid physical contact simply out of fear of causing discomfort to the woman.

There is nothing about breast surgery itself that would require a delay. Even if you still have a dressing, or drains and stitches, there is no reason not to engage in intimate contact. The decision is based more on your emotional state than on your physical readiness.

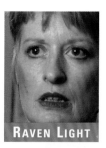

RAVEN LIGHT

I'm a highly sexual woman and so is my lover. I was scared that I would not be able to satisfy her. But my nurse helped us talk the issues out and relearn how to enjoy intimacy.

Often you will have to be the one who opens the conversation about your fears or needs, because your partner may feel that these issues are too personal. Bring the subject up as early as possible. The more time passes without open discussion, the harder it becomes to deal with the issue.

If you're not ready, make it clear to your partner that not wanting to make love is not an act of rejection, and that you may welcome other forms of physical intimacy.

Some women who have had a mastectomy purchase sexy lingerie, or have intimacy in subdued lighting to help take the edge off the presence of a surgical scar, without reducing the feeling of closeness and excitement.

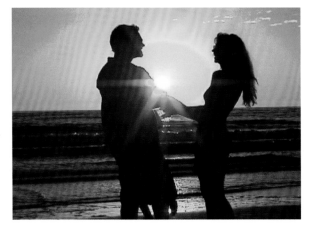

If you have loss of sensation or pain in the breast or nipple area, you may need to gently guide your partner, indicating what is now pleasurable to you.

Hugging, touching, holding, and cuddling may become more important, while sexual intercourse may become less important. Remember that what was true before your cancer remains true now. There is no one "right" way to express your sexuality. It's up to you and your partner to determine together what is now pleasurable and satisfying to both of you.

SINGLE AFTER BREAST CANCER

Being single and trying to start a new relationship, while simultaneously dealing with breast cancer, can add a lot of stress to your life.

The main obstacle is that many women who had a diagnosis of breast cancer feel that they are in some way incomplete or unworthy. "Damaged goods."

I cannot tell you how to begin a successful relationship. But I can suggest the mindset that will guide you at least through the breast cancer issue.

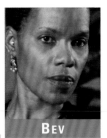

BEV

I never really understood it, but I've had so many... you know, offers... after my mastectomy. I almost think I should have had this a long time ago. It could be men are attracted to my drive to live, because I was faced with an illness that could have caused my death.

The key is to realize that you are not your cancer. You are not a victim. You are not less complete, or less worthy than before your diagnosis. You are who you were. And in addition, as a result of your experience, you are now an even stronger, more interesting, and more understanding person than before. On top of that, the concept that there is something shameful about breast cancer is a thing of the past. It has been "out of the closet" for years! Just check prime time TV programming. Breast cancer is there along with other everyday issues of everyday life.

If you were diagnosed only recently, and the shock is still fresh in your mind, it is difficult if not impossible to be so confident. But have faith—soon your brain will adjust, and you will be able to put your cancer experience in perspective, and realize that it has contributed something positive to you.

How and When do I Tell Him About my Cancer?

One of the challenges is deciding how and when to tell a new acquaintance, who may or may not become a love interest, that you had breast cancer. In Chapter 1 I made a few suggestions on how to discuss your diagnosis with your life partner. But if you are starting a brand new relationship, the question is more complicated. Exactly how and when do you bring up the topic? You are not alone if the thought of informing your date that you are missing a breast makes your palms sweat. As a general rule, mention it early, but not on the first date.

First, how do you say it? If you are uncomfortable articulating the words, there are some tricks that may help you. You've probably heard that some experts recommend that if you are afraid of public speaking, just imagine that the audience is naked. So if you are afraid to say, "I had a mastectomy last year," imagine that your date is jobless, or a diabetic, or Viagra dependent. Now who's got the sweaty palms?

Please understand that I am not diminishing the impact of breast cancer on your life. But it is best to talk about the issue as matter-of-factly as you would about any other difficult experience in your past. And remember: breast cancer, unlike, for example, diabetes, is curable.

How do you decide when, in the setting of a dating situation, is best to discuss the changes that breast surgery might have caused in your body? Many women feel that by clearing the air early on, in the conversational stages, you will be able to relax and enjoy the moment if or when the relationship progresses to intimacy.

As with so many other aspects of the breast cancer experience, you will find that joining a support group consisting of women who are grappling with the same issues, will do wonders for your confidence.

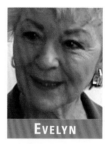

EVELYN

I definitely keep up my social activities. It's one way to fight depression. I go out, do interesting things, maybe even things I've never done before. Push myself a little. I even acted in a medical video!

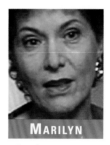

MARILYN

After breast cancer, you're the same person. If you attracted men before, you will attract them after your breast cancer.

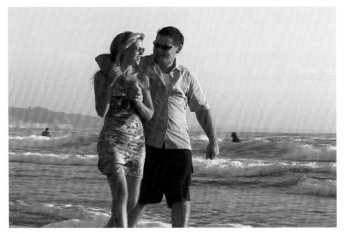

BEING A YOUNG SURVIVOR

Breast cancer is not unique to "older" women. Today there are over a quarter million women living with breast cancer who are under forty. Being a young breast cancer patient presents a number of unique challenges. You are in a different "place" in your life. You might be looking for a date, rather than celebrating a thirtieth wedding anniversary. You may be fresh out of school, instead of planning your retirement party. You may be looking at five decades of life in front of you, not behind you.

It is particularly important for a young woman to insist that her healthcare providers understand her particular needs. Fertility issues may need to be considered in making a treatment choice. Support groups must be age specific. More attention may be given to retaining appearance and regaining sexuality.

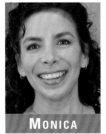

MONICA

I wasn't done with life! I wanted my body to look just as beautiful as it was. I kept pushing my surgeons till we got the result we wanted. And I didn't miss a single beach day, even during reconstruction. Men kept looking ...they couldn't tell I had surgery.

If you are young, take comfort and pride in your strengths. Your body can heal faster. You can tolerate chemotherapy better. And you may be more resilient and adaptable than someone who has been set in her ways for the past six decades.

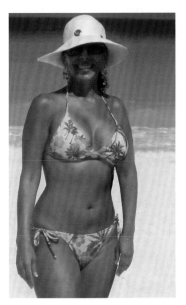

As a breast cancer "minority", a young woman would benefit immensely from interacting with other cancer survivors in her own age bracket. You may want to contact the Young Survival Coalition to get you started. Another excellent resource is PinkLink, a website founded by a young breast cancer survivor determined to help others like her.

NEW BEGINNINGS

New Perspective

The breast cancer experience can be a powerful wake up call to reorder priorities and see life from a different angle. To make a point of finding something enjoyable in every day, in every task. A reminder to stop and smell the roses. Most women report that it has helped them choose new priorities.

Breast cancer can also be a liberating experience. You may decide to do something you always wanted to do—write poetry, travel, or spend more time with your children.

Good Nutrition

This may be a good time to adopt healthy habits. Good nutrition may speed your healing after surgery and help you during chemotherapy. Later on, balanced diet, with proper amounts of protein, fats, carbohydrates, and vitamins will help you feel younger and stay healthier. Currently, there is no evidence that breast cancer can be prevented by a low fat or any other type of diet, although certain diets may affect the incidence of other cancers, such as colon cancer.

Physical Activity

You may have done arm exercises as part of your post-surgical recovery. Physical activity will strengthen and energize you, so don't neglect the rest of your body. A regular exercise program will help you stay stronger and feel younger. There is also evidence that moderate physical exercise can improve the work of the immune system.

Lifestyle Changes

As a breast cancer survivor you may be at an increased risk for other types of cancer, such as ovarian cancer, lung cancer, or skin cancer. This may be an excellent reason to stop smoking and to take better protective measures when you expose your skin to the sun. Other lifestyle changes, such as relaxation or meditation, may help you in your personal and professional life as well. Try to make the whole experience lead you into a better life.

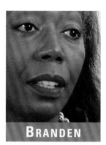

BRANDEN

I started a journal before the mastectomy, when I was first diagnosed with breast cancer. Later, I got a grant from the National Endowment for the Arts, took the journal, turned it into a play, and premiered it at the Los Angeles Theater Center.

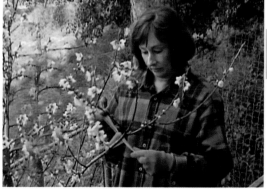

Take the time to smell the peach blossoms

GETTING INVOLVED

As you regain your physical and emotional strength, consider the needs of your fellow breast cancer survivors who may be in earlier, or in more difficult stages of their recovery, and could greatly benefit from someone to guide them through the experience. Many organizations need volunteers who can help other women in their struggle with breast cancer.

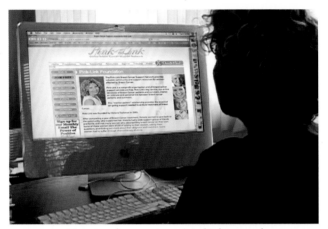

Turning lemons into (pink) lemonade:
Vicki Tashman, creator of PinkLink.org

Whether as a patient advocate who helps mold breast cancer related policy in Washington, a moderator in a local support group, or a helping hand for a friend, you will find that contributing to the cause is an enriching and uplifting experience. A few survivors have started their own breast cancer support organizations to meet a variety of needs faced by women.

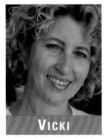

VICKI

I get a tremendous amount of satisfaction knowing that my website, PinkLink.org, helps those women who might feel disconnected to reach toward each other, and stay in touch, and stay informed.

RECOMMENDATIONS FOR YOUR FAMILY MEMBERS

Although the majority of cases of breast cancer are not hereditary, having a first degree relative, either on the mother's or father's side, does increase the likelihood of developing breast cancer. A good word of advice is to inform your family members of your diagnosis, and suggest that your daughters or sisters be particularly thorough in practicing early detection.

The current recommendations include yearly mammograms starting either at age forty, or at an age that is ten years younger than yours at the time of your diagnosis, whichever is earlier.

For younger women, whose breasts are more dense and more difficult to be examined by mammography, ultrasound is an effective imaging technique. MRI has recently been added to the "recommended" list for women at high risk of developing breast cancer.

Mammography is undergoing refinement. For example, a technique called tomosynthesis creates a more detailed, three dimensional image that may be more effective in spotting a cancer, particularly in women who already had cancer surgery.

For younger women, who are not yet at the mammogram screening age of 40 or over, the main tools readily available are clinical breast examinations and monthly self-examination.

Genetic Testing

One of the questions that women who have been diagnosed with breast cancer ask is, "Should my close relatives be tested for breast cancer genes?" This is not a simple question.

The decision of whether to undergo genetic testing should be made with the help of a genetic counselor trained in risk assessment, and the woman must be very clear about the expected benefits and risks.

There are laws that protect patient information, and prohibit health insurance companies and employers from using results of genetic testing to discriminate against a person. But as for anything in the age of online access, there may be a risk that someone may illegally access the information and use it to deny insurance or employment.

The tests that are available today look for abnormalities in a variety of genes. Three of the best-known are BRCA1, BRCA2, and PALB2. Women who inherit a mutation in any of these genes have a much higher-than-average risk of developing breast cancer and ovarian cancer. Your physician or genetic counselor will recommend the right ones for you and your relatives.

If abnormalities are found, then the person may have a higher risk of developing breast cancer. If the test is negative, it does not mean that the person will not develop breast cancer.

For women at high risk, the options include prophylactic mastectomy (removal of both breasts as a pre-emptive measure), or hormone treatment (such as with tamoxifen) that will induce menopause.

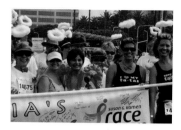

Race by Susan G. Komen

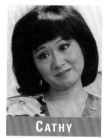

CATHY

One of the most wonderful things about my life after breast cancer is that I've spent a lot of time helping other people. I think breast cancer is a remarkable disease because so many women who are survivors come through that experience and say, "I want to do something to help other people through this."

CHAPTER 14

A GUIDE FOR YOUR PARTNER

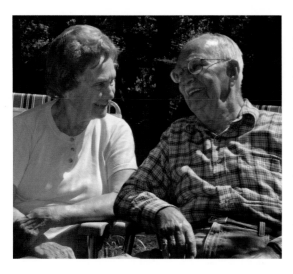

If you had a chance to check the back cover of this book, you probably read that I am a husband of a woman who was diagnosed with breast cancer thirty years ago, and is very much alive and healthy today. Some of the advice I offer in the next few pages is based on that personal experience. The memory of what I went through is as vivid today as it was back then.

As the partner of a woman with breast cancer, you're probably in as much pain and turmoil as she is. The coming days and months will be challenging. You'll have to deal with your own feelings, as well as give the woman you love the support she needs. A positive attitude will help both of you get through the ordeal.

A NOTE ON MY WORDING

To avoid politically correct but clumsy lists of possible relationships, I'll be using "partner" or "spouse" to mean you, the caregiver—whatever your special relationship may be—husband, sister, best friend, life partner, same sex spouse... I'll also use he, she, her or him randomly and interchangeably to avoid the clumsy "s/he" or "him/her" neo-pronouns.

If you can step outside the "cancer" mindset, you will see that this is an opportunity for you and the woman you love to have one of the most rewarding experiences in your life.

WHAT IS BREAST CANCER?

You may know breast cancer as something that requires a big operation and leaves the woman disfigured, or something that is treated with chemotherapy, causing hair to fall out. And something that women usually die of.

In reality, breast cancer that is diagnosed early is one of the most treatable diseases. There has been enormous progress in breast cancer management in the past twenty years. There are effective combinations of treatments that can kill cancer cells, and surgical techniques that give cosmetically pleasing results. In this situation that probably appears pretty dismal to you right now, there are plenty of reasons to be positive.

In the next days or weeks, you should review the appropriate chapters of this book with your partner, and learn with her. Understanding breast cancer and its treatment will help you regain a feeling of control over your life, and will make you a much more effective supporter for the woman you love.

UNDERSTANDING YOUR FEELINGS

"The doctor told me I have breast cancer." These may be the most painful words you'll ever hear from someone you love. Words that bring a flood of emotions—shock, disbelief, confusion—and the inevitable question, "Is she going to die?"

Dealing with these issues is a lot to handle. On top of this, you have an even bigger task. You have to quickly come to grips with your own emotions, so that you can become the main source of support for the woman you love. In the coming days and weeks, you may be asked to play a variety of roles—take notes during medical visits, drive her to chemotherapy sessions, listen without judging, or hold her close when she needs it.

You may feel overcome by the feeling that somehow you must make it all better, and be frustrated when you find out you can't. There is no easy answer, and no shortcut. Accept what you are feeling. Don't be embarrassed. You are facing a serious problem, and it is normal to feel scared, confused, and weak.

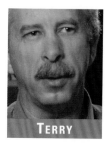

TERRY

I remember hearing a lot from doctors that there wasn't an awful lot you can do, other than hope. I think this is the time when you need to set a direction in terms of your attitude, and build the strength to say, "I'm going to fight this and learn to do what I have to do."

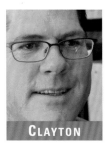

CLAYTON

When Sandy was diagnosed, I just stepped in. I did the cooking – which I hated – but I cooked with my daughter, and I got really good at it. We watched cooking shows together. It gave me a chance to bond with my daughter…

Breast cancer will stress your relationship in countless ways. Your lifestyle will be disrupted—by treatment schedules, or by the new financial burdens that prevent you and your loved one from enjoying your usual activities. The roles each of you played in the relationship may change, and you may find that you are now responsible for tasks that are new to you, or that you are unwilling to tackle. You may have to deal with the side effects of her treatment, such as fatigue, vomiting, or loss of sexual drive. And there will be the turmoil of having to make important decisions while facing the uncertainties of the future.

Fear, anxiety, and sadness will affect how the two of you communicate. Acknowledge these feelings. You can be strong and supportive without holding everything inside. In fact, sharing your feelings honestly with her is the best thing you can do. You may be surprised to find that your loved one appreciates the fact that you can express emotions to her. This sharing improves communication and strengthens your relationship—now, and for the long future.

During the first weeks after her diagnosis you will probably feel like you are riding an emotional roller coaster. There will be days when, after a conversation with your loved one, or a visit to the physician, everything will seem under control, and you will feel strong and optimistic. But that very night, negative thoughts will begin to creep into your head, and you'll feel like all is lost, and there is no hope. You may spend the night pacing, or crying, or wondering what you'll do if you lose the woman you love. By morning you'll remember that there are excellent treatment options, and that her outlook for a healthy life is much better than it seemed a few hours ago. And the world will seem much less gloomy.

These swings of feelings are painful and exhausting, but they are normal. The good news is that with time these emotional tidal waves get smaller and smaller—until they are just ripples in a pond, and you find that you can deal with them.

What Do I Do Now?

If you are like most men, you will probably be eager to put the emotional issues aside, and spring into "action." "OK, so what do I do now?" is probably high on your list of questions. "How do I solve this problem?"

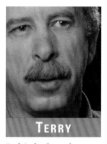

TERRY

I think that the most useful thing a spouse can do for a woman who has just found out she has cancer is assure her that you're not going to walk away and leave her.

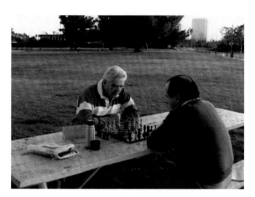

The good news is that you are in a position to contribute greatly to the peace of mind and success of treatment for your loved one. As the husband, partner, "significant other" or principal caregiver, you are in the best position to influence the attitude with which she accepts her diagnosis. And that can make all the difference!

Be as thoughtful as you can in your words and actions. What you do and say in the first few minutes and days after she hears her diagnosis, will make a great difference in how she feels about it herself. Your reaction will play an important role in her physical and mental recovery, so try to be as positive and supportive as you can. One of the most constructive steps you can take is to get involved in her care from the very beginning.

Learn all you can about the disease and the most current treatment options. Search the internet, read books, ask questions. Take the time to discuss the information that the two of you gathered, and compare your impressions. Help her stay focused and not go off on tangents.

Accompany her on visits to her healthcare specialists. Bring a list of questions you want answered. Take notes, or ask for permission to use a voice recorder, so you can review the information you received.

Don't be disappointed by how little you understand at first. First of all, you are listening through a thick curtain of emotional turmoil. Second, breast cancer treatment is a complex topic, and no one can be expected to grasp all the details on the first pass. Trust me on this. I am a doctor, and I understood next to nothing during the first few visits. If nothing else, your mere presence will provide emotional support and a second set of ears.

Questions to Ask Her Doctor:

Do you have any pamphlets or videos about breast cancer we can take home and review?

Is there a Resource Center or patient library in the facility where you practice?

Who would you recommend we see for a second opinion?

Can you put us in touch with women who you treated for breast cancer, and with their partners?

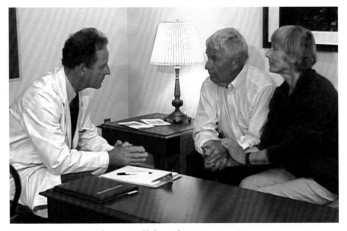

Accompanying her to all her doctor appointments is on one of the most supportive things you can do

If you or your partner feel you need a second opinion, don't hesitate to ask her physician for a referral, or seek one on your own. For something as important as breast cancer treatment, you owe it to yourselves to leave no avenue unexplored. Some of the decisions you two will be making are not reversible, so now is the time to really scrutinize your plan. Don't be afraid to "offend" her physician by asking for a referral to someone else. No reputable healthcare professional will resent your request.

Bear in mind that the diagnosis of breast cancer is almost never an emergency. The few exceptions include inflammatory breast cancer that tends to be rapidly growing and should be treated as soon as possible. In most other cases, you and your partner have several weeks to research your options, and make important treatment decisions. Do not let anyone or anything rush you.

Here is the part that you might find to be the most difficult: you must remember that the final decisions about treatment will be hers. Being supportive and helpful does not mean taking over. If you have been in this relationship for some time, you hopefully have learned when to argue, when to persuade, and when to just step back and say, "Honey, if that is what you want to do, I am here for you one hundred percent."

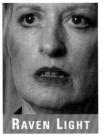

RAVEN LIGHT

Once I was diagnosed, I kind of expected that my lover would just go her way, but she didn't at all. She stayed with me the whole time. From her I learned unconditional love for the first time in my life.

WHAT SHE NEEDS FROM YOU

Emotional Support

Along with the fear of losing her femininity, and possibly her life, what a woman fears most at this time is that you, the one she loves, will abandon her. Emotional support is perhaps the single most important item you can contribute. Knowing that you will be there for her, no matter what, and that you still find her lovable, desirable, and attractive will help her face her diagnosis and tolerate her treatments better than anything else.

You can also help by creating a safe place for her to express her emotions. This means allowing her to grieve in her own way, without making judgments about the "appropriateness" of her behavior.

If you find verbal communication difficult, and choose to hide in your job or in an outside activity, she may perceive this behavior as a withdrawal of your love. Her well being, and the survival of your relationship itself, depends on your willingness to communicate openly. You don't need to make long speeches. Holding her hand, sitting close to her, putting an arm around her, will communicate how much she means to you in ways words can't express.

Most people, especially men, are upset by tearful outbursts, so your first reaction to her crying may be an attempt to "fix it" or somehow "make it all better." But remember that tears are a healthy response. You and she know that there is no easy fix, and to pretend otherwise only delays the grieving that must take place before healing begins.

Anger is also a normal response. Breast cancer is no one's fault, but anger needs an outlet. She may lash out at the closest person during such times. That might be you. The important thing to remember is that despite what she says, she is not angry at you, but at her loss of control over her life. This stage will pass, and she needs to know you'll still be there for her. Help direct that anger into action, to fight against the cancer and depression.

Some women withdraw and refuse to share their feelings, rejecting your efforts at being close. This may be the most difficult reaction to deal with, and may require outside help to re-establish open communications.

Some degree of depression is also to be expected. How do you know if your partner's mood is normal, or if she has a severe depression that requires treatment? This is an important question, because depression can adversely affect her treatment.

It is normal to have short periods of sadness, "blue moods", apathy, or loss of interest in daily activities. You can help her overcome these feelings on your own. But a more serious form of depression, called clinical depression, with prolonged feelings of sadness and loss of interest in all activities, can adversely affect her treatment, and should be managed by a professional.

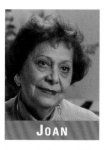

JOAN

There isn't anything that we didn't share. Every word, every feeling, every little thing that went on, we shared. I don't think I could have gone through it without him. He has never said anything that hasn't been, "You're beautiful." And he wasn't afraid to look at the scar and say, "Oh, look how much improvement, isn't that great?" He made me feel wonderful. He made me feel like a star.

- Ongoing sadness and negative statements ("I'm not worth anything anymore." "I hate my life.") lasting a period of weeks rather than days.

- Withdrawing from all normal activities or social/family interactions.

- Physical complaints: sleeplessness or sleeping too much, continual tiredness, over- or under-eating that last a long time.

If your partner displays any of these patterns consistently for two or three weeks, notify her doctor.

Once chemotherapy or radiation treatment is completed, your partner may be overcome with feelings of panic or powerlessness that come from the perception that she is no longer being actively treated. It is important to acknowledge these feelings, then focus on the positive aspects of completing the treatment. There is scientific evidence that a positive mind-set can lead to an improved outcome. A supportive and upbeat attitude on your part will be contagious, and is one of the best ways to help her through the weeks or months of treatment.

A few simple techniques that will improve communications

- Make opening statements that let your partner know you're willing to listen. Comments like, "How do you feel about…" let her know that it's okay to open up on an emotional level.

- Reassure her that she has been truly understood by repeating what you heard in your own words.

- Use nonverbal (body language) techniques to convey how you feel about her. Hand holding, and looking directly at her when she speaks, tells her that your love and concern are real.

- Avoid judgmental comments like, "You shouldn't…" or, "Don't say that." Such statements block true communication by minimizing or invalidating the other person's feelings.

- Be careful with comments like, "Don't worry," or, "Nothing will happen." Having a positive attitude doesn't mean being unrealistic.

- Guys, there is no other way to say it: you just need to learn to be the best *girlfriend* she has ever had. It's OK. Go ahead, be sensitive!

Reassurance About Her Appearance

An unreconstructed mastectomy, or baldness caused by chemotherapy will result in dramatic changes in appearance that will often make the woman feel that her partner will no longer find her attractive. A woman's acceptance of her changed body often depends on your reaction to it. You need to prepare yourself accordingly.

Looking at the mastectomy scar or at the reconstructed breast for the first time can be very frightening. Aside from the change in the familiar look of your loved one, there is the shock of seeing injured skin, perhaps bloody bandages, and drain bulbs full of drainage fluid. If you are at all sensitive to this, it may be a little shocking. But try to keep in mind that once it is healed, the scar will look infinitely better. The swelling, bruising, and bandages will be replaced by a clean white line. Try to be as sensitive and accepting as you can. Give her the type of response that you'd like to hear if you were in a similar situation.

Some women have no trouble looking at the surgical site together with their partners at the earliest opportunity. Others choose to view the scar gradually, sometimes alone, or in subdued lighting, or under the cover of an attractive nightgown. Respect her wishes, and be positive and reassuring when you look at her. What is important is not how her chest looks, but the fact that she is still the same woman you love.

Sexual Intimacy

When is the right time for resuming sexual relations? There is nothing about breast cancer that would prevent intimate contact, even if the dressings and drains are still in place. The deciding factor is your partner's, and your, readiness.

Surgery can be exhausting and debilitating. Tenderness around the surgical site, or loss of sensation in the nipple can interfere with physical pleasure. Wearing a natural-looking prosthesis, or having her partner touch other areas of her body, can help a woman refocus sensation and regain interest in intimacy.

Preoccupation with the cancer and its treatment will probably decrease your and her interest in sexual intimacy. Chemotherapy, in particular, can sap the energy and the motivation out of any sexual relations.

QUESTIONS TO ASK
HER DOCTOR:

Will there be loss of sensation in the breast area?

Will chemotherapy cause her hair to fall out?

Can we see pictures of what the surgical scar could look like?

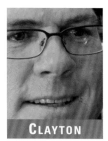

CLAYTON

I initially thought I would have a problem with the change in her breasts. But now – what difference does it make – one smaller, one larger, who cares. Our lives haven't changed, my love for her hasn't changed.

When the time is right, there are a number of small things you can do to rekindle her sexual interest. Make a date with her, give her a foot rub, take a shower together, watch an erotic movie. Try new positions that may be more comfortable. But be patient and know that for many months, perhaps even a year, your sexual interaction may not be the same as it was before.

Help with Daily Activities

After she comes home from the hospital, your partner will have days of physical and emotional exhaustion, and will need your help to handle even the most mundane daily activities. Some women need more help than others. The hard part may be determining how much help she wants. Ask her what she feels like doing on a given day. Look for physical signs of how tired she might be, but avoid "babying" her. Too much help may be as inappropriate as too little. The goal is to return to as normal a life as possible without causing either of you excess stress.

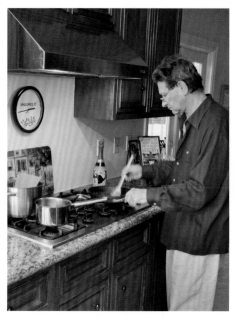

In the early stages of her treatment she may be overcome with a barrage of well-wishing friends and relatives. At first you might feel elated by this, but soon you will find that there is such a thing as too much help and sympathy. You will need to act as the gatekeeper—"well-wisher wrangler" as I called my role. Alternately, you can appoint a specific person to channel all the good-will coming at the two of you.

To avoid alienating friends and relatives, you might want to delegate specific tasks to various people, such as walking the dog, shopping for groceries, driving the car pool, keeping other friends informed, and so on. That way, everyone feels involved, and the necessities of life are attended to. If you have children at home, they will need the time and support your partner may not always be able to give them. One of the most helpful things you can provide is a special time or activity that all family members can participate in—for example, renting a movie or going on a picnic.

You also may be required to deal with financial or insurance issues. There are some things you can do to make an unpleasant task much easier:

- Contact your insurance company at the time of diagnosis to find out their policies on hospital admissions, additional medical opinions, filing of claims and billing, etc.
- Keep a written record of your contacts with insurance company representatives, including names, dates, and times.
- Write down appointment dates and doctors' names. Get a copy of all billing forms, which should include procedures, medications, and supplies used.
- Keep all bills, charges, and related forms together in one place for easy retrieval later.
- Don't forget to keep up insurance premiums. You'll be glad you remembered this critical step later.

MEETING YOUR OWN NEEDS

Finding Support for You

The combination of emotional stress, your regular work, and added activities around the home can take a toll on you. You can't afford to exhaust yourself physically or emotionally. No matter how well you think you are handling the situation, you will benefit both you, and the woman you love, by finding a support person for yourself. A friend, another family member, a religious leader, or a professional counselor who can help you verbalize any feelings and thoughts that you don't want to share with your partner at this particular time.

This support person will help you sort it all out, and work on a plan of action. Talking to other partners of women with breast cancer and participating in support groups can also give you concrete ideas on how to cope. Seeking this form of support for you is not a sign of weakness, but of your wisdom.

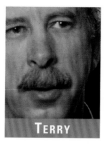

TERRY

It's hard to go and talk to the guys at the office about your wife's mastectomy. I mean, guys just don't open up that much and so there were things that I didn't have anybody to really talk to about. It would have been helpful to have had some support element, whatever it might be.

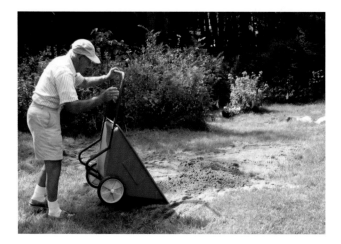

Dealing with the Work

As the primary support person, you will have a major role in keeping up with your family's daily activities during a difficult time. There will be times when you may feel overwhelmed by the entire burden. Before that occurs, sit down with your partner and make plans.

Don't let false pride get in the way of asking for outside help: friends, relatives, neighbors. You can't do it all yourself. If you try, you might use up energy that is best used supporting your loved one.

Planning your workload

• Make a list of tasks that need to be done daily (food preparation, child care).

• Concentrate on activities that really are essential, and put off the unnecessary niceties.

• As people contact you and ask "How can I help?" give them specific tasks that will be truly helpful for you and your partner.

• If you have the financial means, you may want to hire help. Even having someone a few hours a week can ease the situation.

• If you have children, get them more involved in the daily activities. Even young children can be given simple tasks to do around the house, like picking up their toys or setting the dinner table. Actively participating in daily activities gives them a way to cope with their own fears.

MY PERSONAL EXPERIENCE AS THE PARTNER OF A WOMAN WITH BREAST CANCER

Thirty years ago, at the age of 43, my wife went for what we thought would be a routine mammogram of a lump I found in her breast five days earlier. Just as I was starting to realize that she had been gone too long, the radiologist called. "Dr. Lange, we are looking at your wife's mammograms. It looks like she has a malig-

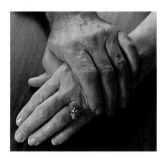

nancy." Just like that. The message was particularly devastating because there wasn't that moment of confusion, that buffer of uncertainty to soften the blow of what I had just heard.

I knew what "malignant" meant. Cancer, mastectomy, chemotherapy, death. I stopped thinking, got in my car, and went down to the radiology facility to pick up my wife.

The most important contribution—sometimes I think it was the only contribution—I made to my wife's recovery, was the attitude I took toward her illness. The thought of being left alone to raise two young children, without the woman I loved, was too frightening a prospect. So I simply decided she was not going to die, and that was that. It was not an option. It was not acceptable. It was my will against the disease, and I was determined to win the battle. In retrospect, we both feel that somehow that mind-set, however irrational, helped make her a *survivor*.

Another, perhaps equally significant form of support was my wholehearted, unequivocal, and immediate assurance to her that I absolutely did not care what form of surgery she may need, and would love her and find her attractive no matter how she looked. Even today, so many years later, she says that it was this attitude that helped her retain her self-image.

In terms of logistical support, "relative wrangling" was definitely a challenge. Both of us come from European families, with their characteristically exaggerated (often grossly exaggerated) response to a diagnosis of cancer. "Oh, my God, how terrible, the poor thing... (read: *she is going to die*). What are you going to do?" To avoid the negative feelings such outbursts would generate, I always tried to paint a much rosier picture of her prognosis, and insisted that no one treat her as a "sick" person.

CHAPTER 15

ADVANCED BREAST CANCER

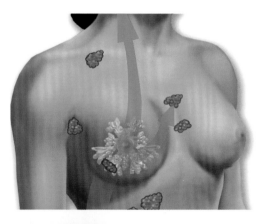

If you were diagnosed with early-stage breast cancer—in other words, if your tumor has not spread to other parts of your body (Stages 0-III) then the information that you need is contained in other chapters. You may safely skip this chapter, which deals with advanced breast cancer.

What is advanced breast cancer? Advanced, or metastatic, breast cancer is cancer that has spread beyond the breast and past the lymph nodes, to form metastases in other parts of the body, such as lungs, liver, brain, and bones. This stage is called Stage IV cancer. About one in ten breast cancers are Stage IV when they are first diagnosed.

Advanced breast cancer may also be a cancer that "came back." In this case, it is also called recurrent cancer.

RECURRENT BREAST CANCER

Sometimes, after the initial treatment, your physician may find evidence that the cancer "came back"—in other words, that you have a recurrence. The recurrence may be local (a small lesion in the breast, along the incision, or near the chest wall), regional (in and around the lymph nodes), or it may be in the form of distant metastases in remote organs of the body. Cancer recurrences usually occur within two to six years after the initial diagnosis, but sometimes even decades later.

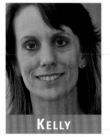

KELLY

It is hard to deal with it the first time. The second time is even harder, but at least you have a better understanding of what to expect. Good thing I didn't throw the wig away.

You will undergo additional testing to make sure that there are no cancer sites elsewhere in your body. The tests are probably already familiar to you from your first encounter with breast cancer. They include MRI, CT, bone scans, and other means of pinpointing areas where cancer may have spread—locally or to distant areas. At that time the decision will be made regarding additional treatment.

A local recurrence will generally be treated with the same approach as an original cancer: surgery, with or without radiation therapy, and possibly chemotherapy or hormone therapy, depending on the size of the tumor and cell grade.

In advanced stages, breast cancer spreads to the lungs, liver, brain, bones and soft tissues. If the recurrence is in another part of the body, rather than in the breast area, treatment will require a systemic approach targeting the entire body. Recurrences that are found in other organs have a much more serious impact on the course of your disease than local recurrences such as those that may be found near the lumpectomy scar.

TREATMENT OF ADVANCED/METASTATIC BREAST CANCER

Sometimes, despite the best efforts for early detection, the cancer is not found until it is Stage IV and it has spread to other parts of the body. The reality of Stage IV cancer (advanced breast cancer and recurrent breast cancer with regional and distant metastases) is that it is usually not possible to remove this cancer completely from your body. Most treatments for advanced/metastatic breast cancer will try to shrink the tumor or to stop it from growing. The good news is that today there are many treatment methods that can greatly improve your quality of life, and extend the time that you remain free of any evidence of the disease.

Surgery

Surgery in the form of a lumpectomy or mastectomy is the key treatment in early breast cancer. But it is not as useful in advanced breast cancer, that presents with metastases outside the breast. If you were diagnosed with a breast cancer that is present in your breast and in other parts of your body, it is possible that your healthcare team may suggest that you forego a mastectomy.

QUESTIONS TO ASK:

Where did my cancer spread?

If it has spread to other organs, is there any advantage to removing the tumor in the breast?

Do you recommend treatment with chemotherapy or radiation to shrink the tumor in the breast?

What tests need to be done on the tumor tissue to find the best treatment for it?

What clinical trials would be best suited to my case?

What support group should I join?

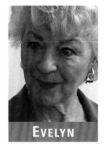

EVELYN

After you cry and rant and rave, then at some point you go, "OK, this isn't going away." And then you can channel your energy into making the very best you can of the situation.

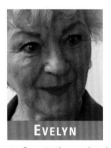

EVELYN

At first Mike and I threw ourselves into the search for a cure. Something had to exist, something western medicine overlooked. Some secret potion? After a while we realized we were just running away from reality.

The reason is that the greatest threat to your health comes not from the tumor in the breast, but from the distant metastases that damage other organs, which generally are difficult to treat surgically.

Surgery may play a role in removing a small, solitary tumor from your lung or liver, or another part of the body where it is applying pressure on another organ. This is called palliative surgery.

Radiation Therapy

Radiation therapy may be used to shrink metastases in distant organs. The treatment will be done by external beam rather than by brachytherapy (see Chapter 6). You may need only a few treatments, rather than the entire five to seven week course.

Chemotherapy, Hormone Therapy and Targeted Therapy

In early cancer, chemotherapy is given to destroy undetectable cells that may or may not have spread through the body, and there is no way to monitor the success of the therapy.

In advanced cancer, your healthcare team may be able to use X-rays or CT scans to observe the tumor as it shrinks from the chemotherapy. If progress is unsatisfactory, the team will be able to switch to another drug, or a combination of drugs. You may want to review Chapter 7 for tips on how to deal with side effects of chemotherapy.

Bones are common first sites to which breast cancer tends to spread. You may be treated with additional drugs called bisphosphonates that specifically target bone metastases, and are given with your regular chemotherapy or hormone therapy.

Hormone therapy as well as targeted therapy can also be used effectively to control the growth and spread of advanced breast cancer. The principles are described in Chapter 8.

COPING WITH ADVANCED BREAST CANCER

It is important for you and your healthcare professionals to be realistic about the probable course of advanced breast cancer. But it is just as important for you to remember that every woman is different, and every cancer runs a different course. Your task now is to avail yourself of all possible resources, and become determined to work toward the best outcome possible.

There are many excellent organizations online that will help guide you on your quest for information. In addition, you may seek out one of several superb books written by women who "have been there before" and who offer their unique insights into dealing with this challenging issue.

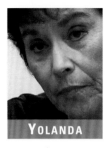

YOLANDA

Remember, at some point docs will only tell you what you ask. So ask. Don't imagine horrors. The truth may not be as harsh as your imagination.

GLOSSARY

abscess
A pocket of pus caused by an infection.

AC
Chemotherapy combination of two different drugs: Adriamycin and Cytoxan.

Adriamycin (doxorubicin)
A drug used to kill cancer cells.

Adrucil (5-fluorouracil)
A drug used to kill cancer cells.

anesthesia
Procedure used to make surgery painless, either by local numbing or by putting the patient to sleep. It is usually performed by an anesthesiologist or a nurse anesthetist.

antiemetic
A medicine that relieves nausea (feeling sick to the stomach) and vomiting (throwing up).

antioxidant
Compounds which slow the deterioration (or oxidation) of cells in the body. Vitamins C and E, as well as beta-carotene are antioxidants.

bank blood
Blood that has been donated and stored for later use.

bilateral
Something that is present on both sides of the body. For example, a bilateral mastectomy is a surgery where both breasts are removed.

blood cell count
A test that measures the number of red blood cells, white blood cells, and platelets in a blood sample.

This test helps evaluate the effect of chemotherapy on the bone marrow where the blood cells are produced.

brachytherapy
A form of radiation therapy in which the source of the radiation is placed close to, or implanted in, the body.

breast form
Something with the shape and texture of a breast, created with tissue or with a prosthetic.

carbohydrate
A chemical compound which serves as a basic source of energy. Foods high in carbohydrates include sugars and starches such as bread and pasta.

carcinogen
Any substance that initiates or promotes the development of cancer.

carcinoma
A form of cancer that develops in the lining of the organs of the body, such as the skin, the uterus, the lungs, or the breast.

carcinoma in situ
A carcinoma that has not spread outside the area where it began.

catheter
A tube used to allow fluid to pass into or out of the body.

cell
The basic building block of all organisms. Individual cells can only be seen when they are magnified through a microscope.

chromosome
One of the many strands of DNA material within the cell that carries genetic information.

circulatory system
The system consisting of the heart and blood vessels which provides blood to all parts of the body.

colony stimulating factors
Chemotherapy additives which stimulate the bone marrow. May be required to maintain adequate blood cell counts during chemotherapy treatment.

combination chemotherapy
Use of two or more chemicals to achieve maximum damage to tumor cells.

cyst
A sac-like structure that contains liquid or semi-solid material.

DCIS
Abbreviation for ductal carcinoma *in situ.*

DNA
Material found in the nucleus of all cells. Contains genetic information for cell division and cell growth.

donor site
Part of the body from which tissue is taken for reconstruction.

double blind
A research study in which neither the participants nor the researchers know which subjects are in the control group and which subjects are in the test group.

doubling time
The time required to double the number of cells in a group of cells or in a tumor. A short doubling time (under 100 days) indicates a fast-growing tumor.

dose-dense chemotherapy
A regimen that uses more frequent administration of chemotherapy.

drain
A plastic tube, usually attached to a bulb, placed into the surgical site to collect any draining blood or fluid for a few days following surgery.

ductal carcinoma in situ
A cancer inside breast ducts that has not grown through the wall of the duct into the surrounding tissues. Also known simply as DCIS.

edema
Excess fluid in a body part. Lymphedema is swelling of the arm as a result of scarring of the lymph ducts after radiation or surgery in the axilla.

estrogen
A female hormone secreted by the ovaries which is essential for menstruation, reproduction, and the development of secondary sex characteristics, such as breasts.

fibroadenoma
A noncancerous, solid tumor most commonly found in breasts of younger women.

fibroid
A tumor composed of fibers or fibrous tissues.

flap
A portion of tissue with its blood supply moved from one part of the body to another. Flaps of muscle, fat, and skin are used to provide tissue for reconstructing breasts.

general anesthesia
Anesthesia which puts your whole body to sleep. Usually given through injection or gases.

genes
Areas on chromosomes that contain hereditary information that is transferred from cell to cell.

genetic testing
Analysis of genetic material (genes) present in *your body*. Certain gene changes (mutations) may predispose you to certain cancers.

genomic testing
Analysis of genetic material changes present in *your cancerour tumor*. Results will help choose appropriate therapy.

guided imagery
Using directed mental images to provide relaxation, mental healing, or higher levels of consciousness.

hemoglobin
A protein in blood which carries oxygen.

HER2/neu
An oncogene which may help determine resistance to hormone and chemotherapy.

hormone
Chemical substance that helps regulate growth, metabolism, and reproduction.

hypofractionation
Administering radiation therapy over fewer weeks, in larger doses.

immune system
System by which the body protects itself from outside invaders or internal defects.

immunotherapy
Therapy that works by enhancing the body's own defense system.

infiltrating ductal carcinoma
A cancer that began in a milk duct and has spread to areas outside the duct.

LCIS
Abbreviation for lobular carcinoma *in situ*.

linear accelerator
A machine that produces high energy X-ray beams to destroy cancer cells during radiation therapy.

lobular carcinoma in situ
A tumor confined to the milk-producing lobules of the breast (LCIS).

margin
The area of normal tissue surrounding a tumor when it is surgically removed.

metastatic cancer
Cancer which has spread beyond the breast to other parts of the body.

micro-surgery
Sewing together almost hair-thin blood vessels with the aid of a microscope.

mind-body connection
A philosophical theory that states that the mind can control bodily functions.

modified radical mastectomy
The most common type of mastectomy. Breast skin, nipple, areola, and some of the underarm lymph nodes are removed. The chest muscles are saved.

myo-cutaneous flap
A section of muscle, fat, and skin transferred for reconstruction of the breast.

needle localization
A procedure in which a radiologist inserts a thin wire into the breast. Later, a surgeon will follow this wire to find the tumor.

neo-adjuvant chemotherapy
Chemotherapy used before surgery, usually to shrink a tumor.

Nolvadex (tamoxifen)
An anti-estrogen drug that may be given to women with estrogen receptor positive tumors.

non-surgical biopsy
A biopsy where samples of a lump or tumor are removed with a needle under local anesthesia.

oncogene
A gene that contributes to the malignant transformation of a cell.

oncologist
A physician who specializes in oncology—a specialty dealing with cancer treatment.

oncoplastic surgery
Use of plastic surgery techniques to achieve both cancer control and pleasing apperance.

oral chemotherapy
Chemotherapy taken in pill form instead of by intravenous injection.

osteoporosis
Increased bone fragility that occurs with age, often due to lack of the female hormone estrogen.

PDQ
Information published by the National Cancer Institute, listing all clinical trials currently underway.

pectoralis muscles
Muscles located under the breast and attached to the chest wall.

port
A device surgically inserted under the skin of the chest, and connected to a very large vein, so that chemotherapy can be injected.

precancerous lesions
Abnormal cellular changes that are potentially capable of becoming cancer.

progesterone
A female hormone produced by the ovaries that causes the breasts to prepare to produce milk.

prognosis
A prediction of the course of the disease; future prospect for the patient.

prosthesis
An artificial breast form worn inside a bra after a mastectomy.

protein
Complex compounds which hold amino acids essential for growth and repair of tissues.

radical mastectomy
Removal of entire breast, as well as underlying muscles, causing significant deformity. No longer performed today.

recurrence
Reappearance of cancer after a period of remission.

risk counselor
A trained healthcare professional who can advise a woman on her risk of developing breast cancer.

saline
A salt water solution,
1. given intravenously during surgery to maintain proper body functioning, or
2. used to fill a synthetic implant for breast reconstruction.

sentinel node
The single axillary lymph node that can be examined to determine if cancer has spread beyond the breast to other lymph nodes.

stem cell
Cells which will eventually become blood cell producers in the bone marrow.

stereotactic core needle biopsy
A biopsy performed using two mammographic views to pinpoint the site of the tumor.

suppressor gene
A gene that can reverse the effect of a specific type of mutation in other genes.

suture
A surgeon's stitch.

tamoxifen (Nolvadex)
An anti-estrogen drug that may be given to women with estrogen receptor positive tumors to block tumor cell growth.

targeted therapy
Therapy that works by enhancing the body's own defense system.

"tummy tuck"
A procedure in which a portion of fat and skin is removed from the abdomen, reducing the size of one's "tummy."

ultrasound
High frequency sound waves used to locate a tumor inside the body. Helps determine if a breast lump is solid or filled with fluid.

visualization
Forming a mental image of something not present to the sight. This technique can be used for relaxation or to help your body fight cancer.

QUESTIONS TO ASK YOUR HEALTHCARE PROVIDERS

The following are questions gathered from the book. They are broken down by chapters with space for your own notes. Feel free to tear or cut out these pages, and give them to the person who will be accompanying you on your medical visits, to use as reminders of what you want to discuss.

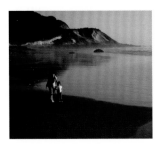

CHAPTER 1: FACING BREAST CANCER

What should I tell my loved ones about my condition?

Can you refer me to a counselor or to a support group specializing in breast cancer issues?

Could you give me the names of specialists you think I should see? How about another set of names so I can choose the specialist(s) I like best?

Is there a multidisciplinary breast cancer team in your facility?

Tell me about your experience in dealing with breast cancer.

Can you give me the name of a breast cancer expert who can give me a second opinion?

Could you forward my chart, test results, and my biopsy slides to the doctor who is going to give me a second opinion?

Where can I find more information about breast cancer? Do you, or your clinic or hospital, have a resource center? A library?

Chapter 4: Surgery

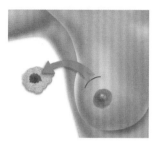

Questions to Ask Your Surgeon:

Is lumpectomy an option for me?   Why or why not?

Does a mastectomy decrease the chances of the cancer coming back?

How will my breast look after the treatment? Can you show me pictures?

Are you and your surgical team experienced in performing this procedure?

Can you refer me to a plastic surgeon so I can discuss my reconstruction options?

What kind of reconstruction procedure do you think would be best for me?

Who can I talk to about my concerns about appearance, dating, pregnancy, etc?

How long before I can go back to my regular activities? Do I need to arrange to have someone help me with my daily activities?

Questions to Ask Your Anesthesiologist:

If I have general anesthesia, how long will it take me to get back to normal?

What will I feel and hear if I have local anesthesia?

Will you give me something to control the pain after I wake up from the anesthetic?

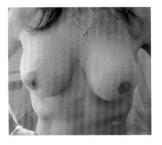

CHAPTER 5: RECONSTRUCTION

Questions to Ask Your Plastic Surgeon:

What type of reconstruction do you think is best for me?

Will an implant make it more difficult to detect a local recurrence?

What should I know about the "skin-sparing" mastectomy?

What is the latest information regarding the safety of silicone implants?

Can you show me pictures of reconstruction procedures you have done?

Could I meet with some of those women so I can see and feel their breasts?

Will my insurance pay for the reconstruction, even if it is done later? Will it pay for a breast prosthesis?

Will I have a lot of pain? How can the pain be treated?

Questions to Ask Your Insurance Company:

Does my policy cover the costs of the implant surgery, the implant anesthesia, and other related hospital costs? To what extent?

Does it cover treatments for medical problems that may be caused by the implant or the reconstruction?

Does it cover removal of the implants if this becomes necessary?

If I choose to delay reconstruction and my company changes insurance plans, will I still be covered for breast reconstruction at a later date?

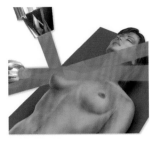

CHAPTER 6: RADIATION THERAPY

Why do I need radiation therapy?

How is the radiation oncologist (physician) involved if the treatments are given by the therapists?

How will I evaluate the effectiveness of the treatments?

Which method is better for me, external beam or brachytherapy?

Can I continue my usual work or exercise schedule?

What side effects, if they occur, should I report immediately?

Will I be able to conceive and bear a child after treatments?

What is the difference in cost between brachytherapy and external beam?

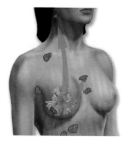

CHAPTER 7: CHEMOTHERAPY

Do I need chemotherapy? Why?

What are the benefits and risks of chemotherapy? How successful is this treatment for the type of cancer I have?

How will you evaluate the effectiveness of the treatments?

What side effects will I experience?

Can I work while I'm having chemotherapy?

Can I travel between treatments (short business or pleasure trips)? What other limitations can I expect?

How can I manage nausea? Should I eat before I come for my treatments?

Will I continue to have my menstrual periods? If not, when will they return?

Should I use birth control? What type do you recommend?

Will I be able to conceive and bear a child after treatments?

CHAPTER 8: HORMONE THERAPY

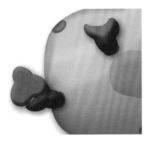

Did the tests on my tumor show that the cells were sensitive to hormones? (Estrogen Receptor Positive, or Progesterone Receptor Positive)

Should I be treated with hormonal therapy or with chemotherapy, and why?

How will it affect my chance to have children?

How will it affect my sexual function?

What side effects should I expect?

Can I get pregnant while taking tamoxifen?

What birth control method would be most suitable to my lifestyle?

CHAPTER 9: TARGETED THERAPY

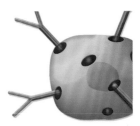

Is targeted therapy right for me?

Would I benefit more from chemotherapy or hormonal therapy than from targeted therapy?

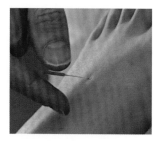

CHAPTER 10: COMPLEMENTARY AND ALTERNATIVE THERAPIES

What benefits can be expected from this therapy?

What are the risks associated with this therapy? Do the known benefits outweigh the risks?

What side effects can be expected?

Will the therapy interfere with conventional treatment?

Will the therapy be covered by my health insurance?

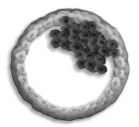

CHAPTER 11: DCIS

What grade is my DCIS?

How well will I do without radiation?

Do you work with a team that includes a mammographer and an experienced pathologist?

What is the downside of getting radiation after removal of the DCIS tumor?

CHAPTER 12: CLINICAL TRIALS

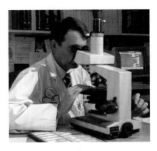

How do I know the facility doing the study is reputable?

Are there other centers doing the same research on the same drugs or methods?

What is involved in terms of tests, treatments, and additional time commitments?

What results can be reasonably expected in my particular case?

What are the currently accepted treatments and how do they compare to the trial?

How can I be sure that I won't be under-treated, or miss the opportunity to be treated with established, conventional therapy?

What would my financial commitment be and how can I cope with it?

Will I need to be available for follow-up testing indefinitely?

Can I travel, work, or move to another city?

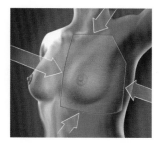

CHAPTER 13: LIFE AFTER CANCER

What can I do if I wake up at night worrying about my cancer?

Will the cancer cells that may have spread to other parts of my body start to grow when I stop taking chemotherapy?

Should my sisters get genetically tested?

Shouldn't we be doing more testing on me to make sure the cancer didn't come back?

What can I do about feeling excessively tired?

Why have I lost interest in intimate relations with my partner?

Why can't I sleep or relax or feel interested in anything?

Why can't I stop feeling that I am going to die because of the cancer?

Chapter 14: A Guide for Your Partner

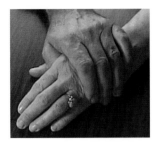

Do you have any pamphlets or videos about breast cancer we can take home and review?

Who would you recommend we see for a second opinion?

Can you put us in touch with women who you treated for breast cancer, and with their partners?

Will there be loss of sensation in the breast area?

Will chemotherapy cause her hair to fall out?

Can we see pictures of what the surgical scar could look like?

Chapter 15: Advanced Breast Cancer

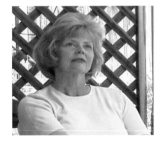

Where did my cancer spread?

If the tumor spread to other organs, is there any advantage to removing the tumor from the breast?

Do you recommend treatment with chemotherapy or radiation to shrink the tumor in the breast?

What tests need to be done on the tumor tissue to find the best treatment for it?

What clinical trials would be best suited to my case?

What support group should I join?

Index

A

acupuncture 102
adjuvant therapy 76, 96
Adrucil (fluorouracil) 88
advanced breast cancer 138-141
alternative treatments 103
anemia 83
anesthesiologist 18, 41, 46-47
anniversary reactions 112
antiemetic 80
antioxidants 22, 98, 101-102
areola 23-24, 45
  reconstruction of 59, 61, 66
aromatase inhibitors 93
arm, caring for 49, 55-56, 116
Avastin (bevacizumab) 96
axillary lymph node 25, 36, 45
axillary lymph node dissection 54
  complications of 54-55
  recovery after 55
  surgical procedure 56

B

biopsy 31, 35
  core needle biopsy 32
  surgical biopsy 32, 34
blood cell count 83, 86
blood transfusions 46
bone marrow 79, 84, 114
bone marrow suppression 84
bone marrow transplant 79
bone scan 35, 36, 114
brachytherapy 69, 73
BRCA1/BRCA2 28
breast
  anatomy and function 23-25
  growth and change 25

breast cancer
  genes 28
  how it spreads 30, 34, 76
  risk factors 26-27
  types 28-29
breast-conserving surgery 6, 39-40, 107
breast implants 57, 59-61
breast prosthesis 68, 133
breast reconstruction 39, 44, 46, 48, 57-68
breast self-exam (BSE) 115-116

C

CAT scan, computerized axial tomography 35-36
check up anxiety 112
chemotherapy 38-40, 49, 67, 71-72, 75-90
  how treatment is given 77-79
  how it works 78-79
  neo-adjuvant chemotherapy 76
  side effects 79-80, 81-85, 87-88
  chemo brain 86
  typical IV chemotherapy day 78-79
children
  dealing with problems 12-13
  help for 12
  telling about your diagnosis 12-13
chromosomes 28, 34, 78
clear margins 42
clinical depression 113, 132
clinical nurse specialist 18
clinical trials 107-110
  how they are conducted 108-109
  is it right for me? 110
complementary therapies 98-103
  mental techniques 99-100
  nutritional techniques 101-102
  other therapies 102-103
control group 108
core needle biopsy 31-32, 34
  ultrasound-guided 32

D

DCIS 104-106

delayed breast reconstruction 59, 67

depression
  clinical depression 113, 132
  reactive depression 111

diagnosis, facing your 7-22

DIEP flap 62-65

diet 27, 101, 123

dirty margins 42

dose-dense chemotherapy 79-80

doubling time 26

drains 48-49

ductal carcinoma *in situ* (DCIS) 29, 104-106

ducts 24
  milk 24
  lymph 24

E

emotional support for you 8, 16-17, 130
  for your partner 9, 128-132

emotional recovery 111

employers 15
  and discrimination at work 15

estrogen receptors 33, 93
  estrogen receptor positive (ER+) 93

excisional biopsy 31-32

exercise 27, 112-113, 123
  after mastectomy 50

expander 60-61

external breast forms 68

F

family
  dealing with problems 12
  telling about your diagnosis 8, 13

fatigue 49, 118
  after chemotherapy 81
  after radiation therapy 72

feelings, understanding your 8, 127-128

fertility 118

5-fluorouracil (5-FU or Adrucil) 79, 88

flap 62-66

follow-up 114

free flap 62, 65-66

friends, dealing with 8, 14, 134

G

genetic testing 28, 33, 125

genetic counselor 18,

genomic testing 33, 76, 88, 89, 125

growth rate 26, 33-34

guided imagery 99-100

H

hair loss 82, 83-84

healthcare team 17-18

hemoglobin 83

Herceptin 33-34, 95-97

HER2/neu 33, 96

herbal therapy 101

homeopathy 102

hormonal therapy 91-94
  how treatment is given 92
  side effects 93-94
  who should be treated 92-93

hormone 91

hormone receptor 33, 91-92
  hormone receptor positive 33

hot flashes 92-94

hot spot 36

hypofractionation 71, 74

I

IGAP flap 65

imagery 100

immediate breast reconstruction 48, 59-61, 67

immunotherapy 95-97

implants, 59-61, 67

infections 41, 55, 67, 84-85
  preventing 85

infertility 118-119

infiltrating cancer 28
infiltrating ductal carcinoma 29
inflammatory cancer 29
informed consent 47
intestinal problems 85
intimacy 119, 121
intraoperative radiation therapy 73
IORT 73

L

Lat flap or latissimus dorsi flap 64-65
laughter, as a therapy 100
life after cancer 111-125
linear accelerator 71
lobe 24
lobular carcinoma *in situ* 29
lobule 23-24
local recurrence 51, 139
local treatment 20
lumpectomy 21-22, 39, 40-44, 52
    and radiation therapy 43, 69-70
    before surgery 41
    is it right for me? 43
    recovery 42
    surgical procedure 47
lymph 23-25
lymph node 23, 49, 53
lymphedema 55

M

macrobiotic diet 101
magnetic resonance imaging (MRI) 35
mammography, after cancer 114, 116
margins 41, 105
mastectomy 39, 45-53
    before surgery 46
    is it right for me? 51
    recovery 48
    skin-sparing 45, 58
    surgical procedure 47-48
medical oncologist 18

meditation 100
menopause 27, 92-94, 118
menopause symptoms, as a side effect 92-94, 118
metastases 30, 52, 75, 138-140
metastatic cancer 30, 139
    advanced 139
micro-surgery 65
mind/body connection 99
modified radical mastectomy 45
mouth sores 27
MRI, *see magnetic resonance imaging*
multi-disciplinary team 16
myocutaneous flap 62

N

nausea 80-81
navigator, nurse 18
needle biopsy, *see core needle biopsy*
needle localization procedure 41
neutropenia 83
neutrophils 83
new beginnings after cancer 123-124
    getting involved 124
    good nutrition 123
    lifestyle changes 123
    new perspective 123
    physical activity 123
    recommendations for family 124-125
nipple reconstruction 66
nipple-sparing mastectomy 62, 63
nuclear bone scan 35
nurse navigator 18

O

oncologist 18
oncoplastic surgery 39
oncoplastic surgery 39, 41, 42
oral chemotherapy 88
Oncotype DX 34, 89
osteoporosis 93

P

Paget's Disease 29
partner
  a guide for your 126-137
  telling about your diagnosis 8-9
pathologist 18
pathology report 34
PET scan 36
pectoralis muscles 24
perforator flaps 65
physical therapist 18
plastic surgeon 18, 57-59
platelets 83-85
ploidy 34
ports
  for chemotherapy 81
pregnancy 25, 27, 88, 93, 119
  and chemotherapy 88
  and hormonal therapy 93
progesterone receptor 32, 93
prosthesis 68
protocol 108

R

radiation oncologist 18
radiation technologist 18
radiation therapy 43, 69-74
  for DCIS 105
  how treatment is given 70
  side effects 72
  treatment planning 22, 70
radical mastectomy 45
RBCs, *see red blood cells*
reactive depression 111
receptors 33, 93
reconstruction 57-68
  delayed 67
  immediate 67
  nipple and areola reconstruction 66
  using synthetic implants 58-60

  using your own tissues 62-66
  which is right? 67
red blood cells (RBCs) 83
relaxation 99
risk counselor 26
risk factors for breast cancer 26
  age 27
  estrogen and birth control pills 27
  family history 27
  menarche 25
  menopause 25

S

second opinion, getting a 16
sentinel node biopsy 56
sexuality 117
  resuming sexual activity 119
  side effects of chemotherapy 79-86
  birth defects 86
  bone marrow suppression 83
  fatigue 81
  hair loss 82
  infertility 86
  mouth sores 82
  intestinal problems 82
  nausea 80
  sexual side effects 86
side effects of hormone therapy -94
  menopausal symptoms 93
  pregnancy 93
side effects of radiation therapy 72
  fatigue 72
  skin changes 72
  other side effects 72
silicone gel implants 59
single women 120
skin-sparing mastectomy 45
social worker 18
spiritual support 100
stages of breast cancer 37

staging 31-33
support groups 17
support network 16-19
surgery 31, 39-56
surgical biopsy 31
synthetic implants 58-61
    silicone gel 59
    saline 59
systemic therapy or treatment 30, 75

T
tamoxifen (Nolvadex) 93
targeted therapy 95-97
Taxol (paclitaxel) 88
tissue flaps 62
TNM, tumor node metastases 36
TRAM flap 62-63
treatment planning 16
treatment group 108
treatment ports 79
tummy tuck 63
tumor testing 33-34
types of breast cancer 28-29
    ductal carcinoma *in situ* 29
    infiltrating cancer 29
    inflammatory cancer 29
    lobular carcinoma *in situ* 29
    Paget's Disease 29

U
ultrasound-guided biopsy 31

V
vascular access device 79
    ports 79
visualization 100
vitamins 101

W
white blood cells (WBCs) 83

Y
Yoga 50, 99

Notes to Self

Consider jotting down something nice that happened today,
or an inspirational quote that appeals to you,
or something you're looking forward to in the next few days.

MY HEALTH CARE TEAM

NURSE NAVIGATOR

_____
_____
_____

PRIMARY

_____
_____
_____

SURGERY

_____
_____
_____

ONCOLOGY

_____
_____
_____

RADIATION THERAPY

_____
_____
_____

APPOINTMENT DESK

_____
_____
_____

NURSE

_____
_____
_____

NURSE

_____
_____
_____

_____
_____
_____

_____
_____
_____